SERIAL HANDBOOK OF MODERN PSYCHIATRY • VOL. I

The Psychiatric Examination

The Psychiatric Examination

JULES H. MASSERMAN, M.D.

Professor Emeritus of Psychiatry and Neurology
Northwestern University Medical School
Chicago, Illinois

AND

JOHN J. SCHWAB, M.D.

Professor and Chairman of Psychiatry
University of Louisville School of Medicine
Louisville, Kentucky

INTERCONTINENTAL MEDICAL BOOK CORPORATION
New York

FOREWORD

Bertrand Russell, mathematician, philosopher and humanist, once remarked "Understanding nuclear physics is child's play—compared to understanding the play of a child." If, then, no single treatise can possibly cover the multiple fields of mathematical physics, it is obvious that no single primer can adequately present the complexities of human personality development, the protean effects of later familial, social and cultural experiences, various interview and diagnostic techniques, multiple tests of neurologic and psychologic functions—and then correlate these interrelated data with disparate systems of psychiatric nosology and prognosis and the almost infinite modes of physical, pharmacologic, dyadic, group, environmental and community therapy. Single-volume texts that attempt this can become superficial, narrowly monothetic or multiauthored conglomerates of conflicting opinions, so ponderous as to be pedagogically forbidding.

To obviate these and similar critiques the authors plan this series of monographs as follows:

1. Each volume will cover the rationale and practices in a sub-field of psychiatry, and can thus be used as a text or reference work for special courses without the necessity of purchasing others not immediately relevant.

2. All will be written as clearly as possible, with illustrative case histories. Cultist jargon will be avoided, or translated into meaningful operational terms either in the text or in an appended glossary.

3. Since the volumes will be published separately, each will be more readily available for early revision as required, and the incorporation of valid developments, than would a single all-inclusive work.

In the above context, this first volume on *The Psychiatric Interview*—the most determinative of subsequent psychiatric transactions—is respectfully submitted to the academic community for use with, and by, students of psychiatry, psychology, social work, nursing and allied fields. Future volumes will deal with child and adolescent psychiatry, clinical nosology and prognosis, dyadic therapies in relation to ancillary group, familial and community modalities, and other topics as indicated by teaching and clinical needs. We hope to be content with whatever acceptance these volumes deserve.

The authors and publisher hereby express their appreciation to W. B. Saunders Company for permission to adapt material from Masserman, J. H.: The Practice of Dynamic Psychiatry. Philadelphia, W. B. Saunders, 1955.

Special thanks are likewise due to Paul Adams, Professor of Pediatrics and Psychiatry, University of Miami, Florida, for Chapter 8, The Psychiatric Examination of the Child. The authors also express their appreciation to Savilla Laird (who also assisted in preparing the Index) and Alberta Berger, their respective secretaries, for their dedication in retyping successive revisions of the manuscript.

Jules H. Masserman, M.D.
John J. Schwab, M.D.

CONTENTS

Chapter 1

PRINCIPLES OF THE PSYCHIATRIC EXAMINATION

There is, generally speaking, no single clinical procedure more important in psychiatric diagnosis and therapy than the assessment of the nature and development of a patient's presenting illness. In order to make this assessment, the examiner must make a directed and thorough survey of the patient's behavioral as well as somatic decompensations, elicit a history of their precipitating causes, assess his past strengths and capabilities as well as his weaknesses and maladaptations, and learn his hopes and fears about the future. After acquiring basic interviewing techniques, the student can develop his own individualized approach to patients, but this should always combine empathy with objectivity and be grounded on a humane, compassionate attitude toward the conditions and dilemmas of human existence. True, the methods and skills involved in this task are difficult to teach by didactic means alone, but with adequate guidance and continued experience, the student soon begins to develop his latent (i.e. "intuitive") knowledge of interpersonal insights and relationships. However, this development may be handicapped by misconceptions the examiner has already acquired about either the objectives or the techniques of the psychiatric interview. Therefore, in order to clear the ground for more positive and fruitful orientations, we shall first review the clinical purposes of the psychiatric examination and then consider some of the misconceptions and impediments.

PURPOSES OF THE PSYCHIATRIC EXAMINATION

The first objective is to confirm the physician's presumably favorable reputation and to strengthen initial rapport. This is accomplished by providing a reassuring milieu for the interview and by adopting a kindly professional manner which will enhance the patient's confidence in the physician's medical competence, friendly interest and wise mentorship. The dynamics and techniques of establishing a therapeutically as well as a diagnostically helpful relationship, beginning with the first interview, will be discussed in subsequent sections.

1

With rapport established, the next objective is to survey the nature of the patient's *current* behavior disorders (the present illness) by an objective, detailed examination of his speech and spontaneous conduct (mental status) and by special tests (physical, psychologic, and other supplementary examinations).

While these may elicit almost every conceivable symptom (variable anxieties, phobias, compulsions, depressions, psychosomatic dysfunctions, excessive drug intake or suicidal preoccupations), the prime purpose is to determine which syndromes are of the most urgent clinical significance.

Third, we attempt to clarify the physical or psychologic stresses that exceeded the patient's adaptive capacities and precipitated the *present illness*.

Finally, as dynamic background and perspective for the above, we investigate the patient's previous *personality*—the characteristic modes of behavior leading to and comprising the exacerbation of the unfavorable patterns under stress, constituting the present illness.

From these preliminary data, we can develop an initial formulation of the patient's problems and disorders both in terms of his conflicts and maladaptations and also of the personal, environmental, and social potentials for resolution. This formulation is based upon a knowledge of the characteristics which were predetermined by heredity, or were shaped by physical development, early formative experiences, or the vicissitudes of later life and an understanding of the biodynamic and environmental stresses inducing the decompensations that brought him to the physician.

IMPEDIMENTS TO THE EXAMINATION

1. The Specialized Approach

The greatest initial handicap often arises from the too limited viewpoint with which students from specialized backgrounds approach their work in clinical psychiatry. For example, the medical student is trained intensively in his preclinical years in the biological sciences and may attempt to base his clinical work in various fields on these sciences alone. Similarly, many graduates in psychology, schooled in formal theory and thoroughly familiar with specialized tests of "intelligence" or "personality," may initially confine their clinical work within the relatively narrow bounds of such concepts. So, too, the social worker, the anthropologist, the sociologist, the young minister faces the danger of approaching the patient less as a troubled human being than as a "subject," "client," or "penitent" to be classified, interpreted, and treated according to some standardized set of preconceptions; indeed, the student who has difficulty broadening his educational and cultural outlook may seek security in a stereotyped cultism which promises simplicity and relief from ambiguities. This can range from an overconcern with irrational, fantastic, symbolic interpretations of all behavior to a categorical rejection of psychodynamic concepts as being at worst unscientific, or at best speculative or irrelevant.

The *exclusively "medical" approach* is a favorite of the physician who, out of anxiety about working with emotionally troubled persons or unconscious hostility toward all "psychiatric cases," is determined to give the patient the "benefit of the doubt" before attaching the supposedly pejorative terms "neurotic" or "functional" to the patient's symptoms. Accordingly, such an interview is taken up with protracted questioning about all physical complaints by organ systems, with full notations as to the nature and results of previous medical or surgical procedures. Usually, there follows an exhaustive physical examination supplemented by a variety of laboratory procedures designed to ferret out some "organic" disease that will bring the patient within the physician's accustomed orientations. True, in many cases this seemingly objective "medical" routine is an excellent device for circumventing the patient's initial anxieties and establishing the necessary belief that the physician is competent and interested in his patient's welfare. Nevertheless, a needlessly prolonged search for organic disease with a concurrent neglect of other possible causes for the patient's difficulties is wasteful, often bolsters the patient's hypochondriacal preoccupations, and sometimes makes it difficult for him to seek advice and help from the physician about his underlying personal problems.

2. The Overemphasis on Deviance

Perhaps the second most common barrier to a complete, meaningful psychiatric examination is the interviewer's relentless search for "psychopathology." As a result of previous training or out of an anxious desire to impress his supervisor, the student may unearth every minute detail about the patient's failures, weaknesses, and aberrations. Such an approach disregards the patient's capabilities and strengths, may shatter his already fragile self-esteem, and may anger and alienate him.

3. Ignorance of Social and Cultural Factors

Another common pitfall is the failure to appreciate that individual maladaptations arise with reference to the special environmental, familial, cultural and social background of the patient. The student, having grown up in a different social setting, may have incorporated many of its values and modalities into his own conception of what is or is not "normal." It is necessary to differentiate between certain behaviors which are subcultural characteristics from those which are symptomatic of "illness." Errors may occur when the examiner has little knowledge about a variety of social and cultural norms and even when he is dealing with patients of the opposite sex or of a different age group.

4. Fear of Loss of Objectivity

Another problem confronting the inexperienced interviewer is that excessive sympathies or aversions for the patient may interfere with obtaining an accurate and complete understanding of his travail. Achieving understanding, intellectually and empathically, while maintaining objectivity, is a crucial problem which must be recognized and resolved by all who work with human beings in distress.

One inadequate refuge is the *questionnaire technique,* whether in the form of case-taking schemata or, worse, sheets of headings and subheadings to which the life story of the patient is fitted with Procrustean ruthlessness. Such forms may be useful in acquainting the beginning student with the types of possibly significant information about the patient, yet they deprive the interviewer of the opportunity to use approaches by which the information can be obtained with the greatest advantage and the least impairment of rapport. Questionnaire techniques, even when they do not flagrantly violate the patient's sensibilities, nearly always render the interview mechanical, superficial, and relatively unproductive, and cannot elicit the rich and infinite variety of human experiences and responses.

Another compensatory procedure is the so-called *nondirective* or *client-centered* interview advocated by Carl Rogers. Essentially this consists of inviting the patient to speak with complete freedom for the prescribed time period without further guidance from the examiner other than occasional and invariably noncommittal expressions of encouragement such as "go on," "mmm," etc. This form of interviewing is a modification of the *free association* technique of psychoanalytic investigation. As such, it is intended to foster a presumably "depersonalized" situation in which the "client" may verbalize his desires, feelings, doubts, and conflicts while the "counselor" acts primarily as a neutral, although occasionally selective, sounding board. However, the rationale for the method takes no account of the covert aspects of human communication, cultural barriers, individual symbolization, and variable interpersonal relationships. Instead, it is based on the sanguine supposition that if only the person interviewed talks freely enough for a sufficient length of time, he will, through presumed processes of "self-realization" and "growth," spontaneously reexplore his difficulties and adopt solutions for them with no "interpretations" or other aid.

However, misconceptions about the "rule of passivity" may result in the avoidance of urgent issues by both him and the patient and may increase rather than diminish anxiety, obsessive-compulsive patterns, regressive withdrawal, and feelings of isolated desperation in patients who have come in urgent need of understanding and skillful help. Indeed, unresponsiveness may be regarded as indifference or frank hostility by persons whose problems are grimly realistic. True, a few articulate patients, long suppressed and isolated, will pour out their troubles best if the examiner, after initial assurances of interest and sympathy, becomes for a time merely a quiet and receptive auditor. Occasionally, a patient will experience considerable relief of tension after such a verbal catharsis, profess gratitude for his "cure," and suspend treatment until his mounting anxiety forces him to repeat the performance. Others may return for infrequent "sessions" over long periods of time, yet continue to verbalize essentially the same stereotyped and sterile ruminations, doubts, ambivalences, and rationalizations. Still other patients--particularly those with strong inhibitions or schizoid and paranoid tendencies--react even less favorably to the lack of feedback in the interview.

Most patients, sooner or later, interpret exaggerated passivity on the part of the examiner as evidence of lack of concern or competence and will seek out someone else who can vary the role of an interested listener with that of a skillful, experienced mentor and guide. In most instances, therefore, the interviewer must make active efforts to enter the patient's universe and communicate with him in a dyadic language before any degree of empathic understanding and rapport can be achieved.

5. A Focus on Personal Interests

A common pitfall for all interviewers is the tendency to lead the patient, directly or indirectly, into a discussion of topics and issues which are of personal interest to the examiner. These may include not only the family or sexual history, but also racial or intergenerational conflicts, religion, special avocations and pursuits or even politics. Sometimes such ancillary discussions reflect the examiner's avoidance of more cogent topics or indicate problems of his own. Or the inexperienced interviewer can be trapped into such discussions by the patient, who thus pleases the interviewer by avoiding more demanding matters.

6. Theoretical or Doctrinaire Preoccupation with the Past

Another pitfall is relative disinterest in the patient's immediate and often urgent problems in favor of unrealistic attempts to explore in fantasied detail his early familial and sexual history in search of "unconscious libidinal fixations," "complexes," or "defense mechanisms" that have ostensibly "governed his behavior at the deepest level" since childhood. Many a patient, although manifestly suffering from grave marital, social, occupational, and even physical disabilities that demand immediate attention, may thus be led into fantasied and unproductive ruminations about remote events in his childhood or even his infancy. An occasional patient may even submit for the physician's delectation an elaborately prepared autobiography detailing supposed "incestuous attachments," "sibling rivalries," "inferiority complexes," and other pseudosophisticated "introspections" and self-diagnoses. Such fantasies may in themselves be pathognomonic of regressive and narcissistic preoccupations, but in these days of overpopularized quasi-analytic literature the patient's initial productions may have no more specific connotation than this.

> For example, an interviewer, after a ninety-minute session with one such patient, reported that he had been able to diagnose "an unresolved Oedipus complex," beyond reasonable doubt, although he had neglected to elicit the fact that his patient had been brought to the clinic by his desperate family because he was a chronic alcoholic and was currently under bond for embezzlement.
>
> Or, on another occasion, a patient with advanced multiple sclerosis denied the organically hopeless nature of his illness and insisted on a psychiatric interview which he opened with the pathetically wishful statement that he knew his illness was "just functional"; thereafter, he plunged into elaborate accounts of early memories, recurrent dreams, "subconscious" wishes, and other such fantasies in the popular tradition of self-analysis.

In effect, these are examples of how both the patient and the inexperienced interviewer, when more or less unconsciously anxious to escape from the troubling real and demanding present, may become immersed in preoccupations about the past which, although indirectly revealing, are often merely a diversion of interest and effort.

7. Covert Hostility to the Patient and Psychiatry

Unfortunately, in a world of insecurities, suspicions, and guarded aggressions, one of the most common ways of reacting to unfamiliar situations is to be resentful of and antagonistic toward those who present them. Rarely, of course, is such hostility to the psychiatric patient expressed directly, yet some physicians almost never use the terms "functional" or "neurotic"—let alone "psychotic"—without pejorative connotations. The hostility toward the patient, covert or overt, may also be accompanied by a derogatory attitude toward psychology and psychiatry. As noted, the examiner may then resort to an exclusively "medical approach" and become preoccupied with drugs and diets for the patient's minor complaints, thus precluding any understanding of the patient's personality problems as the prime goal of the psychiatric interview.

These then, in brief résumé, are some of the pitfalls of inexperience or doctrinal bias—and yet, each has at one time or another been advocated as a methodological virtue. With certain preliminary misconceptions removed, we may now proceed to an objective examination of the content and techniques of the psychiatric examination.

REFERENCES

1. Kallman, F. J.: *Heredity in Health and Mental Disorders.* New York, W. W. Norton & Co., 1953.
2. Rogers, C. R.: *Client Centered Therapy.* Boston, Houghton Mifflin, 1951.
3. Schwab, J. J.: *Handbook of Psychiatric Consultation.* New York, Appleton-Century-Crofts, 1968.
4. Spiegelberg, H.: *Phenemenology in Psychology and Psychiatry.* Evanston, Illinois, Northwestern University Press, 1972.
5. Stevenson, I.: The psychiatric interview. *In* Arieti, S. (Ed.): *American Handbook of Psychiatry.* New York, Basic Books, 1959 (pp. 196–214).
6. Sullivan, H. S.: *The Psychiatric Interview.* New York, Basic Books, 1954.

Chapter 2

RATIONALE OF THE PSYCHIATRIC EXAMINATION

Despite the popularization of psychiatric concepts, even today many patients do not perceive that their bodily dysfunctions and emotional distress may be due to motivational conflicts and failures of personal and social adaptation. For example, the physical discomforts of a peptic ulcer focus the person's attention on his symptoms rather than on the troublesome interpersonal conflicts and other stresses which may produce them; in that sense, the illness can be considered a costly, maladaptive defense against deeper anxieties. The physician may be consulted only after the patient's somatic dysfunctions have exceeded his tolerance, with the expectation that the elimination of their organic cause be the purely medical responsibility of the physician. The primary gains for the patient in such a relationship consist mainly of a diminution of anxiety and emotional conflict; secondarily (epinosically) he also gains solicitude and service from others, relief from responsibilities, insurance compensations, etc.

As a result, most patients are referred to the psychiatrist only after they have made the rounds of other specialists, consulted family or friends, or when their emotional aberrations, obsessive-compulsive strictures or social failures have become excessively disturbing. Moreover, both the referred and those who seek psychiatric assistance directly, usually after pressure by family, employer or friends, continue to hope covertly that their difficulties will yet be attributed to some "nerve disease" or to some easily removable external circumstance.

When referral is resented, the examiner should guard against blaming other individuals (usually a spouse or parent) or imposed stresses as the cause of the illness. Although the patient may obtain some immediate gratification from the feeling that he has an ally or special advocate in the sympathetic interviewer, these tactics eventually fail because they disregard the patient's primary contribution to his own difficulties, and may result in despair about his ever resolving the problem since the fault has been shifted to others or to factors beyond his or the physician's control. Moreover, the patient will later become disillusioned when he realizes that his doctor did not perceive the situation accurately. Instead, (a) a careful inquiry into the nature and development of the patient's symptomatology

8

may indicate quite clearly the neurotic nature of the disorder and also its covert determinants, (b) positive information about the dynamics and the patient's difficulties is yielded by his behavior in the interview and during the physical, neurologic, and laboratory examinations, and (c) these reassuringly objective approaches relieve the patient's initial anxieties and suspicions, bolster his confidence in the physician, and so eventually permit him to discuss his personal difficulties more directly when he is encouraged to do so. The medico-psychiatric approach useful in the majority of cases may be didactically outlined as follows.

The Setting

The examining room should be intimate, quiet, comfortably furnished and not glaringly illuminated. Certificates confirming the interviewer's professional qualifications should be unobtrusively displayed, as may autographed photographs of former teachers or other items which likewise modestly testify to his status and competence.

PRESENTING COMPLAINTS

After a cordial, reassuring introduction designed to set the patient at ease, invite him to state in his own words what symptoms or complaints led him to seek psychiatric help. His statements in this regard may, of course, cover a wide spectrum, ranging from a complete denial of any difficulties (e.g., "I don't think there's anything wrong, Doctor; the boss [wife, friend, et al.] just sent me for a check up.") through categories of a variety of physical or intellectual impairments (e.g., "headaches," "difficulty with concentration," "frightening thoughts") to direct confessions of drug addiction, growing despondency, or suicidal preoccupations. Such statements are always significant, but often they are primarily evasive gambits not only vis-à-vis the examiner but also toward significant others in his life, and usually constitute only one expression of more pervasive difficulties. For example, the patient who states that "nothing is wrong" may continue to use such denials (as he does at home and at work) until he regards the examiner as a completely trustworthy and potentially helpful person. Other patients focus almost exclusively on discrete physical complaints as open or thinly veiled challenges to the psychiatric examiner as a competent physician until the patient is willing to explore the concurrent emotional aspects of the illness. Or patients who immediately begin with a direct outpouring of "confessional" material may at first become excessively dependent and later covertly hostile when the physician, instead of fulfilling the omnipotent, all-benevolent role, sooner or later points out that the patient himself must change some or many of his cherished but impractical ways. It is generally well, however, to postpone such directives until mutual respect, rapport and confidence have been gained.

With these initial therapeutic relationships established, the examiner may begin to probe tactfully beneath the usual denial, vagueness, or circumlocution of the patient's initial communications. In the beginning, this probing should take the form of requests for more specific information about the exact nature, dates and circumstances of the origin and development not only of the patient's presenting complaints but also of all other symptomatic disturbances. Such questioning, far from arousing resentment, further reassures the patient of the physician's interest and diagnostic thoroughness. Thus, focused inquiry can be made regarding the symptoms characteristic of anxiety states, depression, obsessive-compulsive behavior, psychobiological disturbances, and other syndromes readily detectable by their clinical expressions. Indeed, this portion of the examination may yield sufficient information to make possible a fairly accurate preliminary diagnosis. One caution, however, must be carefully maintained: namely, that the patient, even in his description of apparently specific symptoms, will continue to employ some vague, euphemistic and ambiguous terms unconsciously designed to hide rather than reveal the neurotic aspects of his behavior. Some of the patient's presenting complaints—the predominant symptoms which ostensibly have driven him to seek help—include physical dysfunctions, general manifestations of emotional distress, or direct expressions of concern about a "neurosis"or a "mental disease." Typical complaints which require further clarification are as follows:

Physical Complaints

Pain

Pain is probably the most common symptom of distress, mental or physical. Pain is used by patients as a legitimate complaint by which they gain access to physicians. It may be used to obtain sympathy or attention or to disguise feelings of grief or aggression. "Psychic pain" has limitless associations; for example, trauma, deprivation, grief, unfulfilled eroticism, disillusioned satiation, or expiative punishment.

Certain questions are helpful in eliciting the full import of the pain. What produces it? What relieves it? What is it associated with: set times or activities, in what situations, alone or with whom, in fantasies or in dreams? What does the patient do—obtain medication, rest, relief from strain? Is it a covert device for not meeting supposed or real obligations? What do others do when the patient has pain? In essence, what are its manifold meanings to the patient and to the significant others in his life?

Headache

Complaints of headache may refer to actual cephalalgias ranging from mild dyesthesias to torturing hemicranias, and must, of course, be investigated from the standpoint of a possible ophthalmic, meningeal, toxic, or other organic etiology. Much more frequently, however, an offhand complaint of "headache" can be shown on objective inquiry to refer to quite other varieties of experience: e.g., sensations of muscular tension in the shoulders and back of the neck that are common in anxious patients; feelings of general heaviness, dullness or oppression, common in melancholics; or states of boredom, pique, impatience, and irritability that have made the plea of headache a traditional though thinly veiled excuse for escaping undesired social obligations.

In many, the complaint of headache seems to symbolize concern about adequacy, about difficulties in coping, or fears that one's mental capacities are overtaxed. For example, many students complain of headache and difficulty in concentration as they describe the increasing demands made upon them; and many of the underprivileged, particularly young black women in their 20's and 30's, complain of headaches which appear as a manifestation of their struggles to integrate their family relationships in the face of uncertainties and oppression. A simple symptomatic inquiry into what the patient means by "headache" and an outline of its formal characteristics (time of onset, duration, method for obtaining relief, etc.) may reveal that it is more often the result of emotional distress or of neurotic struggle than of organic disease.

Dizziness, Faintness

Such complaints may have their connotations of vertigo, ataxia, weakness or syncope; more frequently, however, they are used to cover reactions of anxiety, depersonalization, sexual excitement, confusion, impending panic, and other subjective states of widely diverse psychiatric significance. An exact description of what the patient implies by such terms as "jitteriness," "buzzing in the head," or "blackouts" may elicit information relevant to a differential diagnosis of purely "functional" disturbances of consciousness as distinguished from Meniere's disease, episodic hypoglycemia, pyknolepsy, epilepsy, or other substrates for the episodes of impaired awareness. Attention to the timing of the onset, the interpersonal or other situation in which it occurs, and measures for alleviating the symptom may provide significant information about the patient's basic conflicts (e.g., aggressive, sexual or other interpersonal dilemmas) and characteristic modes of reactivity (e.g., avoidance behavior or hostility).

Complaints Related to Anxiety Reactions

Relatively few patients will directly admit experiencing periods of irrational fear or anxiety; or in their account of such episodes, they will conceal the fantasies and conflicts which precipitate them. Instead, they complain of sudden "attacks" of chest pain, weakness, shortness of breath, "butterflies in the stomach," tingling in the extremities, etc.—symptoms of sympathetic nervous system discharge and/or hyperventilation—which they interpret as impending "heart failure," a "stroke" or imminent physical calamity. Such episodes sensitize the patient to the degree that he becomes unusually aware of normal bodily functions which he then continually monitors. Complaints of a "racing" or "pounding" of the heart may refer to sudden vivid awareness of quite normal heart action. Other symptoms such as "hot flashes" may mean only extreme uneasiness; "choking" may denote characteristic anxiety-engendered sensations in the throat; "pains in the stomach" may inaccurately describe abdominal tension; or "fluttering in the stomach and fainting sensations" may refer, not to splanchnic constriction, muscular weakness or clouded consciousness, but to diffuse or overwhelming apprehensiveness. Preoccupation with and the monitoring of normal bodily functions or the symptoms of tension states then become the focus of the patient's concern, obscuring his awareness of conflicts, stresses or interpersonal difficulties. So defined, the patient's reactions are then pathognomic of a recurrent *anxiety syndrome* which may range in intensity from mild phobic reactions to catastrophic disorganization as well as serious hypochondriacal states.

Other Somatic Complaints

An objective, disarming, and unprejudiced inquiry may further indicate that various bodily dysfunctions are related to conflicts, stresses, and failures and differ from those caused by organic lesions alone. In general, neurotic symptoms are diffuse, protean and variable, and are influenced in form and in severity by the emotional state of the individual; therefore, they become manifest in particular environmental or social circumstances. For example: symptoms of ulcer, chest pain, or fatigue may appear only when the patient is working at resented tasks; the introverted recluse may experience urinary frequency or generalized itching at a social gathering; or the immature insecure wife may develop vertiginous or fainting episodes when she feels alone or uncertain of protection by her husband and family. The "body language" of physiologic dysfunctions may be eloquent: i.e., overeating and obesity can often reflect "oral" needs for dependency and love; nausea and vomiting may represent unconscious reactions of distaste or disgust; indigestion, diarrhea or urinary urgency may express inner uneasiness or rejections; and, amenorrhea and constipation may be part of a generalized depressive inertia and psychomotor retardation. Such symptoms are tacitly accepted by the patient as an integral aspect of his efforts to adapt when needs are not met and conflicts go unresolved.

"Mental" and "Nervous" Complaints

Complaints of "Nerves" "Nervousness," "Nervous Exhaustion," or "Nervous Breakdown"

These are prime examples of the popular euphemisms often used by the patient and other informants to connote any and all forms of distress and behavior, ranging from mental anguish to overwhelming fears, or from mild idiosyncracies to behaviors indicative of psychosis. The popularity of such terms is understandable: they are vague enough to be noncommital, they are socially acceptable, and they may carry a connotation of organic causation; however, they have no specific psychiatric meaning whatever, and should not appear in the case record except in a direct quotation such as, "the patient's presenting complaint is that he has 'felt nervous for about a year.'" Unless this statement is defined and further elaborated, it is as though a physician obtaining a medical history stopped with the patient's initial plea that he "felt sick," instead of proceeding to elicit a further description of the exact nature, intensity, localization, sequence, duration and present status of the patient's symptoms.

The common complaint of "fear of a nervous breakdown," too, has a wide range of personal meanings. Sometimes the patient uses it to try to convey that he is overwhelmed by life's demands and is unable to cope; or it may express a patient's fears that he will lose control and openly act on his sexual and aggressive impulses—i.e., become exhibitionistic or flagrantly assaultive. To other patients it means helplessness and fear of possible institutionalization, and to still others, it means occupational or marital or social failure and disgrace. A tactful, skillfully directed inquiry into the meaning of a complaint such as nervousness will then elicit a clearer symptomatic description of current or past states of tension or anxiety, distortions of affect, obsessive-compulsive or phobic behaviors, or even more serious schizoid deviations. Throughout the interview, the patient's terminology must be specifically interpreted within wide latitudes of meaning: for instance, the complaint of recurrent "fears" may refer to realistic apprehension, to neurotic phobias, or to paranoid fantasies, whereas "fixed ideas" may range from obsessive ruminations through preoccupations with wishful fantasies to schizoid delusions. Which of these interpretations is to be placed upon the patient's initially vague descriptions of his behavior is obviously of the greatest diagnostic and prognostic import.

Complaints of "Neurosis"

One other and more recent type of presenting complaint deserves mention: namely, increasing numbers of patients consult the physician or psychiatrist with the "frank" complaint of being "neurotic." Here at last, it may be thought, the physician can proceed to a direct examination and analysis of the patient's personality, but this may not be the case. For in a large number of instances, the patient may use the term "neurosis" not to indicate any meaningful recognition of his problems, but as a convenient blanket under which to hide his real difficulties in personal and social adaptation. Some patients wear their "neurosis" as a somewhat anachronistic but shining armor designed to the latest fashion and emblazoned with their private crest, behind which they feel safe enough to deal with the world on their own terms. Nor is this armor loosened when the patient, for devious reasons, consults the physician; indeed, the prognosis for making his defenses unnecessary is considerably less promising than in cases in which the patients are neither so blatant nor so well-organized. The following cases may illustrate some of these clinical problems:

CASE 1. The self-styled "intellectual" who, having dabbled in Freud, Adler, Rogers, Korzybski or Berne, has already "explained" his own "neurosis" in terms of his "libidinal fixations," his "inferiority complex," his "alienation," his "semantic referents,"his "childhood" and so on, and merely comes to the physician ostensibly to confirm his erudite formulations so that he can continue his presumably unalterable patterns of behavior, however destructive they are to himself and others. When an attempt is made to induce such a person to face his maladjustments and responsibilities in more realistic terms, his usual response is to seek another physician whom he can more readily instruct in "depth psychology," "semantics," "transactional analysis," etc.

CASE 2. The thrill-seeking woman of means who, bored by her routine and generally futile existence, becomes intrigued by the fashionable and romantic possibilities of being "psychoanalyzed."

CASE 3. The ne'er-do-well son of an overprotective family who is sent by them on a round of physicians and psychiatrists for advice and recommendations which are tangentially purchased and never followed.

CASE 4. The patient who comes with a pathetic trust that the magic of psychiatric guidance can somehow help him surmount realistic economic, social, or even physical stresses. The latter category now includes an increasing number of patients who, misled by lay misconceptions of "psychosomatic medicine," seek psychotherapy as a last fond hope of cure for chronic, advanced, and essentially irreversible somatic diseases.

A pitiable instance of this was a cultured, highly intelligent, 27-year-cld engineer with a fulminating case of nephrotic hypertension who rejected the hopeless prognosis given him by three expert internists, insisted that his physical disabilities were entirely "neurotic," and clung to the idea that if he were treated by psychoanalysis—for which he was willing to pay any fee—a complete cure could be affected.

Complaints Indicative of Depression

Many college youths or disillusioned middle-aged patients complain that they are tired and sad, that life has lost its zest, and that the future appears bleak and gloomy. More frankly depressed patients present complaints ranging from localized aches in any part of the body to diffuse tension, fatigue, and various physiologic dysfunctions such as loss of appetite and weight, or episodic over-eating, indgestion, constipation, delayed or fitful sleep, early awakening, hypersomnia, morning fatigue, loss of sexual interest or complete frigidity or impotence. The patient may appear to be mentally and physically retarded or he may be restless and agitated. Often only the patient's furrowed brow, lines of tension on his face, flattened tones, and sagging musculature betray his sadness and his melancholy mood, which is thus communicated to the examiner by his appearance and mimetics rather than by verbal description.

Depression is known for its many masks. The patient with the "jovial depression" can be particularly difficult to recognize: a middle-aged man who wears a fixed, tense smile which conceals underlying sadness and despair. Only after rapport is established can the interviewer begin to sense, indeed to "feel," the grimness behind the facade. Many of these patients are especially high suicide risks; they live with desperation and some have already determined on suicide unless a concerted effort to alleviate their depression succeeds.

SUPPLEMENTARY INQUIRIES AS TO THE SYMPTOMATOLOGY OF THE "PRESENT ILLNESS"

Thus far, we have analyzed only the patient's presenting complaints and have seen that, whereas they are inevitably informative, when contextually understood, they are mainly significant as an initial statement of the behavior patterns to which he consciously wishes—perhaps misleadingly—to direct the examiner's attention. Obviously, these complaints do not represent the whole of the patient's "present illness," and must therefore be supplemented by a comprehensive inquiry designed to elicit other and perhaps more significant aspects of the presenting clinical problem.

Here again, an analogy with the general medical interview may be instructive. A diagnostician, confronted with a patient's primary complaint of "pain in the abdomen" first obtains as much information as he can about the onset, location, quality, intensity, duration and course of the pain, and then proceeds to a full and pointed inquiry as to other symptoms in relation to the physical functions of the entire body. This is done for the obvious reason that even a well-defined abdominal pain can be just one part of many diverse syndromes, whereas the same presenting complaint becomes pathognomonic if it is associated with other symptoms of gall bladder or appendiceal disease, peptic ulcer, heart failure, peritonitis, ureteral calculus, or other clinical entities. Apparent, too, is the fact that many patients cannot give a coherent account of the various symptoms that constitute these conditions unless they are helped by an objective but carefully directed inquiry by a physician familiar with the syndromes of the pathologic conditions which he seeks to diagnose and exclude.

So also in the psychiatric examination, the first objective is to determine which phenomena are within the range of normality, which are manifestations of neurosis, or which are the more severe and possibly bizarre symptoms of psychosis. This evaluation of symptoms requires an adequate description of their nature, variation, interrelationships and present status. A detailed account of the onset of the symptoms, their relationship to altered circumstances (e.g., change of work or vocation, divorce, pregnancy), the effects of medical as compared with mainly suggestive "therapy" (e.g., chiropractic or faith healing), and the immediate reasons for consulting the psychiatrist may in themselves demonstrate the character and the meaning of the presenting dysfunctions. A more specific and detailed consideration follows:

Anxiety

Many consider anxiety as the affect which engenders maladaptive neurotic and even psychotic deviations of behavior. In neurotic reactions, the anxiety may still be felt and expressed directly or it may be partially obscured by phobic, compulsive, regressive, or other manifestations. In the psychoses, anxiety may emerge in naked, terrifying form (e.g., overwhelming panic, fears of dissolution and impending doom, etc.), or it may be

concealed behind deep melancholy, irrational euphoria, or highly personalized, variably bizarre ideas of persecution or unreality which reflect the
fragmentation or disorganization of the personality.

Indirect symptomatic expression of anxiety consists of (1) *subjective
symptoms*—a sense of apprehension and fright; (2) *psychophysiological
concomitants*—shortness of breath, palpitations, feelings of constrictions in
the throat (globus), nausea, muscular tension, tremor and restlessness. A
surprisingly large proportion of "functional" complaints are, thereby,
manifestations of chronic neurotic anxiety or of mixed depressive conditions. The circumstances that precipitate and those that relieve these symptomatic expressions yield important clues about the relationship of the
patient's neurosis to familial, sexual, occupational, social, or other stresses
and conflicts.

Obsessions, Compulsions and Phobias

A stereotyped routine of living is a common defense against anxiety in
our insecure, highly competitive society. To a certain extent, therefore,
intensive preoccupation with life's problems in an effort to find realistic
solutions may be of value. However, when ruminations become repetitive
and circular, and result merely in stereotyped, unproductive patterns of
behavior, the effects may become seriously deleterious. Many deprived and
underprivileged persons admit to "having to do things over and over again
to make sure they are right" as a compulsive way of trying to cope with the
complexities of the poorly understood technological world; they hope for
some degree of acceptance and approval as "slow but able" workers.

Depressive Reactions

When there is a sense of pervasive sadness underlying the presenting
complaints, the interviewer should ask directly about the patient's dysthymic mood and his capacity for enjoyment. Such questions may lead the
interviewer and the patient to a discussion of losses, real or symbolic,
which preceded the onset of his condition, the patient's reactions and his
diminished security and self-esteem.

Many of the symptoms of depressive illness vary with the patient's
social class. Early in the course of the depression, the relatively well-to-do
patient's presenting complaints usually consist of loss of interest in social,
occupational and even recreational pursuits. The middle-class patient's
symptoms tend to be characterized by sadness, crying, fatigue, irritability,
and a sense of inadequacy and helplessness. Economically or culturally
deprived patients complain of feelings of futility, pessimism, and hopeless-

ness. Usually, depressed patients, regardless of class, also seek medical relief for disturbances of appetite and digestion, sleep, and sexual activity —which are revealed when the interviewer questions the patient about them.

Severely depressed patients, particularly adolescents and young adults, and white men in their 50's and 60's, are high suicide risks. Therefore, as soon as it is appropriate to do so, the interviewer should ask the patient frankly and tactfully, but without using any evasions or circumlocutions, about how often he thinks about suicide and whether he has changed his will or insurance program recently. Fortunately, most depressed patients respond favorably to the interviewer's willingness to open up this subject; they interpret his concern as evidence of his capacity for understanding and desire to help. This may include acceptance of immediate hospitalization to protect both the patient and the physician against fatal diagnostic oversight.

Intake of Drugs and Alcohol

Many patients are dependent upon tranquilizers or antidepressant medications, or irrational combinations of them, which have been prescribed by physicians, which they have obtained by borrowing from well-intentioned family or friends, or which they have bought at the local drug store in response to reprehensible advertising. So also, housewives may use "diet pills" routinely as mood elevators without being aware that most of the drugs in this group are amphetamines which can become habit-forming deliriogenic and somatically injurious.

Many patients are already addicted to barbiturates, alcohol, tranquilizers, or other drugs before they are referred for or seek psychiatric evaluation. Drug abuse cannot be viewed solely as an aspect of the "youth culture" or "counter culture." In some form, it prevades all age groups and social levels. A large number of patients will attempt to conceal from the physician, consciously or unconsciously, the extent of their drug use and dependency. Therefore, it is essential that an account of such drug intake, including prescribed and over-the-counter medications, form part of the investigation of the present illness. This is necessary in order to assess the possible toxic effects of drugs and is certainly mandatory before other medication is prescribed. Moreover, information about the patient's drug use—types of medication, frequency of usage, when and how obtained—provides valuable clues in a short time about the nature of the person's disturbances (e.g., diet pills used to counteract depression), its severity, and the situational stresses involved (e.g., tranquilizers before the executive board meeting or the housewife's "upper" pill or a "stiff drink" just before the husband comes home).

How the patient obtains the medication sheds light on his willingness to seek aid or his need to "go it alone." For example, some patients rely excessively on physicians to mitigate the problems of everyday life by imploring, persuading, or even demanding prescriptions, often from a number of different doctors. Such tactics enable the patient to avoid confronting his problems directly. Other patients, who medicate themselves with over-the-counter drugs, may fear that, once disclosed, their problems, like the miseries from Pandora's box, will prove to be so overwhelming as to shatter the pretenses and denials they use to make life bearable.

Few persons seek help because they have been using marijuana, and focusing on it usually provides little information that is of value for the psychiatric interviewer. Fears about marijuana impel some parents to coerce their teenage children into therapy after a series of clashes which result in the teenager's feeling insecure, conflicted, and even "neurotic." During the initial session the interviewer will have to delve intensively into the intergenerational problems, the parents' often exaggerated fears, and the fundamental reasons for the teenage patient's lowered self-esteem and impaired self-concept, rather than focus on the topic of marijuana.

Recently, young patients have voluntarily sought psychiatric assistance because of unpleasant deleria during "bad trips" on psychedelic drugs, and fear that they have been harmed by their use or by addiction to "uppers" and "downers" in various combinations. Generally, these patients first complain of difficulties in concentration, fatigue, problems with parents, and about the futility and lack of direction in their lives. After a few minutes, however, as soon as they feel that they can trust the interviewer, they will freely describe their drug use, particularly if they are questioned about it in a quiet, simple, nonaccusatory manner. Even those who blatantly announce that their problem is "drugs" use this as an opening gambit to obtain help, often not for their drug intake per se, but for feelings of anxiety, depression, unreality and confusion.

The misuse of alcohol is probably the most common drug problem in the United States and in other countries throughout the world. Many people who refuse to define themselves as alcoholics are unable to go through the day without drinking much more than they admit to themselves and to others. Appropriate inquiries about how much, when and in what circumstances the patient imbibes can determine the extent of his reliance on alcohol and indicate situations which he perceives as threatening or stressful. Simple questioning about whether the patient thinks he "drinks too much for his own good" may open up a frank discussion of the over-use of alcohol and its interpersonal and other complications.

Regressive Behavior

The survey of the present illness should include preliminary notes about the extent to which the patient has relinquished social duties and responsibilities, adopted patterns of excessive dependence or exaggerated invalidism, and accepted secondary gains (often at the expense of other family members) such as preemptive care, protection, or financial compensation for his "illness". The patient is likely to conceal, consciously or not, the fact that in many ways his behavior affords him devious ways of escaping responsibilities or of expressing covert aggression against his parents, spouse, employers, physician, or others toward whom he is motivated by covert hostilities. There is little to be gained at this time by belaboring the point of whether the patient's behavior in these respects is unconsciously neurotic or deliberately calculated (i.e., malingering) since in many respects the distinction is in itself a spurious one. Instead, the tactful interviewer should obtain information about the patient's diminished desires to function at various levels, his interpretation of the impairment, and the reactions of family members and others. This part of the survey may be of considerable prognostic import; if overprotection, unearned sympathy and other secondary gains are too readily provided or the patient's regressions have become fixed, the prospects for effective therapy are correspondingly diminished.

Schizoid Tendencies

The presence of progressive introversion, isolation or even more ominous schizoid tendencies must be ascertained and evaluated. Such symptoms may include: (1) mild feelings of unreality, (2) unusually frequent lapses into fantastic reveries, (3) affective distortions manifested by exaggerated or by unusually flattened emotionality, (4) illogical or bizarrely symbolic thinking, (5) inappropriate or deteriorated social conduct, (6) delusional (dereistic) misinterpretation of time, place, sequence, and significance, and (7) paranoid, diffusely destructive or other manifestations of frank psychoses. When such symptoms become apparent during the interview, they should be confirmed by questioning the family or other physicians. Sometimes, however, out of the need to "protect" the patient from any implication of "insanity," the family will have overlooked the nature and gravity of the patient's aberrations or will be loathe to describe objectively what they have observed.

Cautions

From the preceding, it is evident that an account of the patient's "present illness" will furnish a fairly adequate appraisal of the nature and severity of his symptoms, and will also indicate the type and character of the environmental situations that precipitate or alleviate them. However, the psychiatric examiner must acquaint himself with the richness, variety, and differential significance of neurotic and psychotic behavior and learn to use this knowledge to detect patterns of illness.

CASE 5. As another clinical instance, if a patient complains of a recurrent migraine, further inquiry even of a superficial nature may reveal that his headaches occur regularly every weekend that he spends with his wife and family, whom he perceives as nagging or boring, that the pains disappear when the patient regains the haven of his work on Monday morning, and that they are rarely troublesome when the patient is on a solitary vacation. True, these circumstances are not determinative, since the headache may conceivably be due to fumes from a furnace at home, to allergic reactions to the roses in the patient's garden, or to other such remote possibilities. Much more likely, however, the migraine is a symptomatic expression of marital and familial conflicts, and even has an adaptive function in that it affords the patient a compromise escape into quiet, protective isolation, while at the same time, with ostensible innocence and suffering, he makes the rest of his family tread lightly and give up other interests to nurse him. This interpretation would be strengthened by knowledge that physical and laboratory findings were normal, that previous medical treatment had given only temporary relief, that the headaches were accompanied by other presumably psychophysiologic symptoms (e.g., anxiety, obsessions, compulsive behavior), that all of these symptoms had first appeared at about the time the patient began having familial conflicts, and that symptomatic improvement had occurred during periods of separation or of reconciliation.

The patient's description of his present illness may also reveal that he has recurrent and obsessive fears of "some day forgetting myself and hurting my family," that he has developed an aversive ritual of not handling knives, that he now sleeps and eats alone, and that he has come less for treatment of his hemicranias than for assurances that recent vivid nightmares of violence and murder "do not mean that I'm going insane and may not be able to control my actions." Such data would justify the tentative diagnosis of an anxiety-ridden, severely obsessive-compulsive individual with migrainous reactions to emotional stresses probably related to marital, familial and sexual conflicts. Of course, determination of complicating organic factors in the patient's neurosis, more searching interpretations of the dynamics involved, and an analysis of the patient's personality development would still require further data.

At this point, however, another word of caution should be inserted about the danger of prematurely ascribing disturbances directly to specific emotional stresses on the basis of anamnestic evidence alone. Every person's lifetime is almost inevitably marked by repeated disappointments, frustrations, and conflicts, and these may or may not play a significant role in precipitating response patterns sufficiently aberrant to be termed neurotic. In this connection, particular care must be taken in making diagnoses on the basis of circumstantial evidence; the mere concurrence of symptoms in relation to emotional stresses does not "prove" the etiologic role of the latter.

CASE 6. Consider the example of a young man referred for psychiatric care with a preliminary diagnosis of "nervous dermatitis." On questioning, this patient readily revealed that two weeks previously, while on a beachside picnic, he had proposed to a girl and had been turned down. He had become despondent, lost his appetite, couldn't sleep, daydreamed at work, and two days later developed a severe macular eruption for which he had been sent to the referring physician. With such a history, it might justifiably be inferred that the patient experienced a reactive depression related to his severe disappointment in love; however, one cannot also conclude that the skin rash was a "neurodermatitis" related to the emotional trauma. The rash might have been more directly caused by poison ivy or delayed reactions to insect bites at the picnic, in which case the interrelationship of dermotoxic and neurotic factors would also have to be evaluated. The itching may then have contributed markedly to the patient's insomnia, and the patient, during wakeful nights of lovesick rumination, may have further aggravated his skin condition by preoccupied scratching. In many instances, such intercurrent causes can disconcert the hasty and unwary psychiatric diagnostician and handicap effective therapy.

The principle of the overdetermination (multiple influences on interrelated emotional reactions and symptoms), illustrated perhaps too simply by the preceding case, must be considered in all so-called "psychosomatic" disorders. Thus a diagnosis of neurosis, although on adequate criteria, is insufficient for designating *all* of the patient's complaints as neurotic, since often a more careful clinician—or ultimately a pathologist—may demonstrate that this did not make the patient immune to a ruptured gastric ulcer or a fatal disease. On the other hand, the physiologic disturbances that accompany anxiety states, depressive conditions, and other neurotic reactions may contribute to irreversible pathologic changes in various organ systems that reach dangerous proportions requiring specialized medical and surgical care.

THE ENVIRONMENTAL BACKGROUND

Heretofore, we have been concerned with the clinical appraisal of some of the most urgent aspects of the patient's present illness—the physician's first task in the psychiatric examination. Nevertheless, however accurately the physician may discern the nature and development of the patient's symptoms, he must remain continually aware that he is dealing with a human being living in the here and now under "real" circumstances. The patient's "reality," of course, is as *he* conceives it, but for this very reason, the patient-milieu relationship constitutes an indivisible "biosphere" (Angyal) which must be respected and dealt with as an operational entity. No survey of the "present illness" is complete without knowledge of the patient's background, his marital state, family responsibilities, occupation, economic status and other data that translate an abstract "case" into a unique living person in his particular social setting. Even a few minutes devoted to gathering these essential sociodemographic data yield an abundant supply of meaningful information: e.g., the patient's annual income, occupation, and educational level indicate highly significant past and present strivings and stresses. Nevertheless, a man with only a high school education who has risen in the business world by dint of constructive planning, financial shrewdness, and dedicated work, may be lacking "status crystallization," and be socially troubled about the seeming lack of congruence of educational, occupational, and income levels.

CASE 7. A 50-year-old farmer with a 10th grade education accumulated large land holdings near an expanding resort area, began building resort hotels, and within a few years was the owner of a chain of motels and recreational businesses. With the new wealth his life style changed dramatically. But he developed first a peptic ulcer, and later, serious disabling tension headaches for which he was eventually referred for psychiatric treatment. Poignantly, he confessed that he was lonely and friendless. In the country club circle to which he now belonged, he felt ill at ease because he used bad grammar and could not converse with the "elite." And he was no longer welcomed by his former fishing companions who used flimsy excuses to exclude him from their expeditions. Moreover, his socially conscious wife and young adult children, who were comfortable with their new life of luxury, either ridiculed him or embarrassedly apologized for him in public.

CASE 8. Or consider, for example, the case of a highly educated assistant professor whose income is not commensurate with his intellectual achievements and who has to contend for years with the everyday stresses of genteel poverty.

Information about parental occupation and income provides knowledge about upward and downward social mobility. Exceeding previous familial levels of attainment may induce guilt, anxiety, and resentful reactions toward the parents, all of which can combine to engender conflict and interpersonal difficulties with other parental figures. Conversely, if the son or daughter of successful parents does not equal their achievements, the failure is incorporated into the patient's self-concept, and may become manifest in negativism, alcoholism, neurotic dysfunctions, and social rebellions.

As noted, the interviewer must also perceive what is considered normal and abnormal in the different ethnic, social, economic, or religious groups with which the patient identifies—information which is vitally necessary in order to view the patient's reactions and symptoms in their proper perspective.

> For example, with the migration of various groups from the Caribbean to the United States and the massive rural-urban shift, beliefs in witchcraft, hex, and voodoo are now common in the ghetto areas of our large cities. These patients frequently present bizarre symptoms such as paralyses, respiratory disturbances, and spells of syncope or "dropping out." Some racial groups fear the revengeful return of the spirits of dead parents, and may experience frequent and severe anxiety reactions. In such cases, an especially tactful, reeducational approach, with the cooperation of ethnic healers, must be employed to provide symptomatic relief.

PRECIPITATING CIRCUMSTANCES

An account of the occurrences in the patient's life that led most directly to the need for medical or psychiatric consultation is always useful. Many patients are referred for psychiatric care after a variable period of unsuccessful medical or surgical therapy. As we have seen, such patients may still be convinced that their illness is organic and are either covertly resentful or are at least poorly informed about the purposes of their referral. In many of these cases, the patient would not have come at all had not various external influences forced his decision. These may include impending loss of a job, threats of divorce, or pressure by family members who have become either overtly condemnatory or reactively oversolicitous.

Precipitating events cover the entire spectrum of human experience, and their clinical importance depends not on the examiner's preconceptions but on the patient's unique interpretations of their significance. As but one example, a death in a family may tragically incapacitate one person but appear as a liberating event to another.

OBJECTIVES

The patient may, at first sight, appear to be consciously subversive. He may have come to the physician with the express purpose of securing a letter to his employers stating that the strain of "overwork" or the "shock" of a recent near-accident had caused a "nervous breakdown" for which he

wanted financial compensation. The tremendous increase in traffic accidents and resulting litigations, and the large number of malpractice suits
tend to involve more and more physicians and psychiatrists in legal maneuvers to obtain financial benefits for alleged physical or "nervous" sequelea.
The ethical physician is likely to recoil from the more or less conscious
dishonesty of many of such requests, and may reject the patient outright as
an unprincipled self-seeker or "malingerer" undeserving of the psychiatric
advice and help which is extended without reservations to the "genuinely
mentally ill" person. Nevertheless, even those frankly seeking financial or
other material compensations may have deep-seated character difficulties
which brought them indirectly for help; their immediate purposes differ
only in degrees of frankness from those of other patients. Rare indeed is
the patient who comes for "therapy" with more than fragmentary insight
that his neurotic behavior is neither necessary nor to his best interests.
Instead, many patients more or less consciously wish only to be aided in
removing what they perceive as "external" obstacles and frustrations to
their happiness.

> Eric Berne points out that the most common of *Games People Play* is: "If It
> Weren't For You." This captions, for example, the exceedingly common marital
> situation in which one partner lives with the fantasies about the joys and happi-
> ness which would be realized if only the spouse were not an obstacle. Such
> patients frequent physicians' and psychiatrists' offices, usually seeking con-
> firmation of their views—professional support which, if hastily supplied by the
> inexperienced interviewer, will be used by the patient only for self-vindication
> and further attacks upon the spouse.

THE PAST HISTORY: THE STUDY OF PERSONALITY DEVELOPMENT

As has been indicated, the initial survey serves to define and in large part
to clarify the patient's "presenting illness." Nowhere in modern medicine,
however, is there any such entity as a disembodied "illness" and the psychiatrist, too, must always keep in mind that he is dealing not with "mental
diseases," but with a *person* whose characteristic patterns of behavior,
"normal," idiosyncratic, or "abnormal," have been formed long before
recent accentuations of the latter patterns brought him in for medical or
psychiatric aid. Indeed, as the physician gains a deeper understanding of
the multiple dynamic factors that determine the continuity as well as the
vicissitudes of human conduct, he will be less able to demarcate sharply his
patient's presenting illness from the increasingly maladaptive deviations of
behavior that preceded and conditioned it. This applies even when the phys-

ical and environmental "precipitating traumata" are severe (e.g., as in toxic confusional states or combat neuroses), since the central problem will remain; how did the patient come to be especially susceptible so that inter-current stresses could induce the array of decompensations and aberrant responses that constitute his disabling "present illness?"

Obviously, these questions can be answered only by investigating the patient's "personal history"—not as a mere chronological account of the events in his life but as a well-directed and insightful analysis of his cultural and familial background, his physical endowments, his childhood environment and his scholastic, sexual, occupational, social, and other formative experiences. With such data, the physician can reconstruct the patient's development: the genetic potentials and the experientially developed motivations, attitudes, sensitivities, talents, symbolisms and patterns of behavior that characterize him as a person and that form the substrate for the "illness" the physician is called upon to treat.

Sources of Past History

Information about the patient's life can obviously be obtained from many informants, though most conveniently and significantly from the patient himself. It may be argued that autobiographical data, however skillfully sought and truthfully offered, are very likely to be selected and distorted to accord with the patient's repressive amnesias, wishful fantasies and varible attitudes toward the interviewer. And yet, this seeming dilemma has a pragmatic aspect, namely, that irrespective of what the "facts" were, (and what human account is other than "subjective") *the patient's own interpretations and evaluations of his experiences* have far greater psychiatric significance in most instances than any ostensibly "objective" biography furnished by others—especially since the latter accounts, too, can only be compendia of remembrances, opinions, and judgments which generally reveal more about the respective informants than they do about the patient. When specially indicated, supplementary data can also be obtained from school, institutional, and employment records, and from reports of medical consultants, though all such testimony must be weighed in accordance with the biases and personal interests of the observer.

With these interpretations and reservations, we may now proceed to consider the customary *organization* of the anamnesis.

The Family History

This is usually taken as a description of the patient's antecedents and close relatives, and was considered highly important in the days when hereditary factors were thought to play a paramount role in the etiology of mental disorders. As has been indicated, however, data obtained from the patient about the family forebears or others is chiefly useful as an index of his own attitudes toward the persons he is describing.

> CASE 9: A not unusual case is one in which a patient characterized his father as selfish, harshly domineering, and a "hellion when drunk," whereas the patient's sister described the same father as considerate and lenient, driven to take an occasional drink only when the patient's own behavior became intolerable. These descriptions obviously furnished little "objective" information about the father; nevertheless, they served the more significant purpose of indicating with considerable clarity the status of various interpersonal relationships and attitudes within the immediate family circle.

When a patient describes a parent in completely unambivalent terms, either as a thoroughly despicable person without any redeeming virtues, or as a saintlike figure devoid of faults, he displays not only biases and fragmented views, but also his incapacity to live with the ambiguities and uncertainties of adult human relationships. When a patient begins to remember, for example, that his mother whom he had previously characterized as "completely rejecting" had really spent many hours comforting him during an illness, he is beginning to live with more flexible attitudes toward himself and others.

In the same way, descriptions of more distant relatives are, of course, subject to even greater distortion through personal bias or selected hearsay —a fact often neglected in questionnaire studies of presumed "hereditary factors in nervous and mental diseases." Nevertheless, it is useful to record descriptions from various sources as to the occurences of mentally retarded, neurotic, sociopathic or psychotic behavior in the direct or collateral heredity of the patient, provided such data consist, insofar as possible, of descriptions of specific behavioral deviations, records of institutional care, medical diagnoses, and similar relatively objective evidence. However, for the transactional evolution of the patient's behavior, it will generally be sufficient to secure adequate characterizations of the patient's parents and siblings, supplemented, if possible, by his impressions of relatives (particularly grandparents), nurses, governesses, teachers, or other parent-surrogates who may have exerted formative influences on his life. Similarly, it will be illuminating to record personality descriptions of the patient's spouse, children, co-workers, or other individuals who play an important role in his current relationships in various spheres of activity.

Childhood History

It is manifestly absurd to expect the patient to remember exact details of his behavior during infancy; in fact, any specific information he offers in this regard is mainly significant in indicating narcissistic preoccupations either with tales about his childhood relayed from the accounts of parents or siblings, or else with ready-made pseudoanalytic formulations derived from reading or previous consultations.

Recollections of vivid childhood experiences may also be offered by the patient; such "screen memories," although generally quite inaccurate as to time, place, and events, are nevertheless significant as symbolic representations of important events in childhood which he distorts and pictorializes and thereby "screens" in both senses of the word.

CASE 10. As an example, a 35-year-old housewife sought psychiatric consultation because she feared that her sexual coldness would drive her newly successful businessman husband into the arms of his attractive secretary. While recounting salient facts about her early childhood pertaining to the number of people in her home, ages of siblings, etc. she suddenly gasped, broke into tears and murmured that she had been afraid of penises since her 19-year-old brother-in-law had fondled her and made her masturbate him when she was only 5 years old. She later embellished this story with such lurid details that it became impossible to distinguish fact from fantasy. In effect, exaggeration of this ostensible "childhood trauma" really epitomized her repugnance toward all men—an attitude basic to her sexual problems.

Similar "screening" of purported early memories and the way in which both the recalled and the omitted events relate to present complaints should also be kept in mind while gathering data on the following points.

Birth and Early Development

The parents' ages and the quality of the marital relationship at the time of the patient's conception may be significant. Was the patient a wanted child? By which parent? If the patient was conceived in order to "save the marriage," was he or she used as a pawn in the marital game during childhood or later life? Or, if the mother was pregnant before marriage, was the patient regarded as an instrument of bondage which coerced the parents into a life together with him as the principal victim? Recollected information as to complications of pregnancy and delivery, early illnesses, length and routine of feeding, weaning difficulties and approximate ages of sitting, walking, talking, and sentence formulation ("normal" ranges: ±4, 9, 12, and 18 months respectively) may also be significant with regard to mental and neurological impairments when they exist. Adolescent or adult neurotic patterns may sometimes be traced to early feeding disturbances, or problems manifested by excessive crying, persistent thumb sucking, enuresis, incontinence, scoptophilia, night terrors, tics, spasms, phobias, temper tantrums, or unusual cruelty or destructiveness. Other topics which may be of significant value include early selective attachments or aversions to parents or siblings, the types of disciplinary training and habit development, and responses to familial stresses. In particular, the patient's attitudes toward siblings and especially the birth of younger children in the family should be elicited.

Schooling and Early Socialization

The pertinent information about these important subjects involves the age at which the patient went to nursery school, kindergarten, and grade school, the type of school (public, parochial or private), his readiness to leave home, and his responses to teachers and schoolmates. The patient may be asked about which subjects he liked and disliked, and what his grades were; in addition to such rather simple data, information should be gathered about possible school phobias, truancies, resistances and delinquencies. Most patients respond freely to direct questions about whether they enjoyed or disliked schooling and the extent of their participation in play, sports, and other activities, particularly those which involve cliques, clubs or group loyalties. Such a survey from kindergarten through the grammar grades will reveal the patient's strengths, talents, and potentials as well as possible reactions of anxiety, shyness, and aggressive competetiveness or schizoid or other tendencies.

Later Personal History

This should begin with the time the patient enters junior high school and is approaching puberty. Many patients tell that their first difficulties occurred in the immediate preadolescent years when they had difficulties forming significant peer relationships. The history of this life period is designed to reveal the further modifications or crystallizations of behavioral patterns and neurotic or psychotic tendencies under the social, sexual, occupational or other stresses of adolescence and adult life. The data may be recorded under the following headings:

Sexual Development

When approached objectively and openly, almost all patients will discuss their sexual development; in fact, it may be necessary to limit verbose

and detailed accounts of childhood, adolescent or later sexual ideas and
fantasies from patients who still cherish a popularized notion that all neuroses may be traced to early sexual experiences. As is true of most of the
personal history, the patient's account of early erotic fantasies, curiosities,
inhibitions, and even activities will undoubtedly be distorted by later experiences; but, for the very same reason, his "recollections" will reveal much
about his present attitudes. The information about sexual development
should consist of data about the age at which—and how—he or she became
aware of sexual drives, knowledge and cautions about such activity,
events regarded as "sexual traumata" during childhood, age of menarche,
attitudes towards masturbation, and type and degree of other erotic outlets. Screen memories of witnessing intercourse between parents (so-called
"primal scenes") or accounts of childhood seductions may be fact, fantasy
or a mixture thereof. Social repressions, inhibitions, and "castration fears"
may also be deduced from the patient's denial of masturbatory experience
or his anxiety and guilt about them.

The interviewer should inquire about dating, social concerns, adolescent
infatuations and "crushes," preference of and emotional reactions to various sex partners, the circumstances and frequency of sexual arousals, relative continence or promiscuity, sex techniques and pace, and the repressions, overcompensations, sublimations, and other defenses the patient
employs to ease his or her sexual anxieties and conflicts. Particularly indicative of the latter are excessive hesitations, jealousies, doubts and ambivalences during premarital courting or periods of engagement. The marital
history should note the occurrence not only of impotence or frigidity, but
of lesser degrees of delayed, premature or disturbed orgasm, the choice of
and adjustments to birth control measures, suppression or satisfactions of
extragenital erotic desires, reactions to conception and childbirth, and
other sexual tensions and satisfactions. If this information has been secured
by proper anamnestic techniques, the patient will proffer similar and even
more confidential data regarding marriages, separations and divorces, and
extramarital temptations, adventures and experiences.

In the past, in view of the stringent taboos on homosexuality and
"perversions" in our culture, the interviewer had to be especially cautious
in inquiring about such tendencies or practices; however, with increasing
knowledge and changing mores, patients expect simple, frank, unembarass-
ing questions about homosexual play or activity. Even if at first denied,
homosexual tendencies may be deduced from other familial, occupational
and social relationships.

Personality Traits

The development of patterns of diet (including fasting, food fadism or
periodic gastrointestinal orgies), dress, sleep, recreation and other modes of

conduct is of psychiatric import either when they become neurotically compulsive, or so culturally deviant as to interfere seriously with the patient's social adaptations. Specific inquiry should be made as to the patient's recommended or self-prescribed intake of cathartics, "tonics," "vitamins" and other medications, as well as his degree of indulgence in tobacco, tea, or coffee, or his addiction to alcohol, marijuana, sedatives, barbiturate derivatives, demerol, and other drugs.

Secondary School and Higher Education

The familial, economic, and personal determinants of the choice of schools and curricula are significant, and specific abilities and deficiencies are indicated by success or failure in particular studies. The scholastic record should also be evaluated from the standpoint of selective interests, later relationships with teachers and mentors, acceptance or rejection of discipline, and the evolution of goals and responsibilities. Similarly, information about the joining or organizing of clubs, participation in extra-curricular sports or cultural interests, and the patient's status in various school groups furnish other significant indices of his developing personality patterns. Against this background, premonitory neurotic, dysthymic or schizoid trends may appear as first evidences of serious difficulties in personal and social adaptation.

Occupational History

Information about the choice of work, constancy and intensity of application, the types of success attained, and the reasons for changes or failures reveals a great deal about the patient's strivings and capacities to utilize talents and accept limits. The patient's reactions to group discipline, his ability to cooperate with others, tendencies to overwork or to avoid unpleasant routines, and possible periods of enforced idleness should also be evaluated. Particularly significant are his occupational prides or aversions, and his characteristic reactions to what he regards as successes or failures.

Later Social Adjustments

These comprise the types and constancies of friendships cultivated, the general gregariousness or isolation of the patient, and the extent of participation or leadership in religious, volunteer, fraternal, political or other group activities. Under this rubric may also be placed information about adult hobbies or interests, recreational preferences and practices, and special circumstances that lead to a sense of social failure. Additional data may then be secured, as indicated, about the patient's prejudices, social objectives and ethical or religious convictions as reflected in his daily living.

Adjustments in Later Life

As will be seen in later clinical discussions, the fifth and sixth decades of life may bring problems that overstrain the individual's capacities for adaptation. Long-cherished ambitions must be regretfully surrendered; children mature, become emancipated and drift away; physical vigor, sexual attractiveness and erotic pleasures wane; occupational, economic and social inadequacies grow imminent; and, life may seem to hold little in prospect but a bleak and insecure old age. Under such stresses a great variety of excesses and self-indulgences may be developed to deny advancing age. These include attempts to hold the family group together by querulous dependency or authoritarian demands for allegiance; impulsive sexual liaisons, divorces and remarriages; injudicious investments or business ventures in desperate efforts to achieve economic security; hypochondriasis with devious attempts to restore lost youth by medical or surgical means; and excessive religiosity or spiritualistic preoccupations. If and when these fail, reactions of anxiety and dysthymia occur; these range from variable moodiness to sweeping and persisting despondencies which are variously and often misleadingly labelled "menopausal depression" or "involutional" or "presenile" melancholia.

MEDICAL HISTORY

While obtaining the personal history, the interviewer should question the patient about illnesses, accidents, and surgical procedures during early and late childhood, adolescence, and adult life. The presence of disease—its type, duration, severity, treatment, and degree of invalidism—should be related to the developmental phase or period of life at which it occurred. Recurring episodes of illnesses indicate special vulnerabilities and tendencies to react with the same symptoms to a variety of physical or psychosocial stresses; e.g., some patients are gastrointestinal reactors who develop nausea, vomiting, or diarrhea as the earliest symptom of any illness or as a response to problems or stressful situations. Moreover, painful or prolonged illnesses during early childhood, for example, not only traumatize the child, but also determine his attitudes toward disease and health care in later life.

Information about such illnesses reveals a great deal about the quality of the parent-child relationship. A mother's overly protective concern about the child's health may restrict his or her participation in sports and other activities and impair normal social development. Overweening parental care may lead the patient to expect this from others as his right when he becomes ill later in life. Conversely, the parent's exhorting the child to endure pain and suffering stoically, may lead to the denial of illness in adulthood or to the overreactive rejection of a spouse who does not attend to all the patient's needs for care promptly.

When a patient gives a history of recurrent illnesses, the interviewer should always inquire about the incidence of the same type of illness in other members of the family, particularly parents. Repeatedly, patients who give histories of recurring symptoms such as headache, sore throat, gastrointestinal distress, or asthma, will, when questioned, report that a parent was frequently incapacitated by similar illnesses, as illustrated by the following case vignette.

> CASE 11:   A 26-year-old woman sought psychiatric assistance because her erratic work record was causing trouble between her and her student-husband who was dependent upon her income. She was unable to work regularly because of frequent sore throats (diagnosed occasionally as mild, nonspecific pharyngitis) which she had had since childhood. Questioning revealed that when she was a child, her mother had "gone to bed with a sore throat" at times of stress. The mother's repeated illnesses, described as life-threatening "strep" infections, dominated the family life and were apparently used to manipulate family members, avoid obligations, and secure attention. When the patient realized that her illnesses were patterned and that antibiotics were now available in case she developed a really serious infection, she began to explore more satisfactory means of coping.

Importantly, it is necessary for the interviewer to find out what physical illness, and particularly surgery, meant to the patient at the time and what fears and fantasies persist. Abdominal or perineal surgery during adolescence may be perceived as a sexual attack which is accompanied by fantasies that continue to influence symbolic attitudes toward sexual activities. One patient may wish to believe that a minor facial scar resulting from an accident is the severe cosmetic disfigurement responsible for his social unpopularity. Another patient may heedlessly disregard actual limitations produced by disease or injury and jeopardize his health by excessive physical activity or endanger the lives of others by insisting that they accompany him in these activities.

From the medical history, therefore, the interviewer can glean critically important information about the patient's responses to physical stress and his attitudes toward physicians and family members. His reactions may include hypochondriasis, regressive invalidism, denial of illness, distrust of physicians, dependency on medical care, excessive demands on family members and other deviant patterns. Merely listing physical diseases, surgical procedures, and hospitalizations is insufficient if it does not bring to light the special meaning and the enduring effects of each episode or reveal tendencies toward accident proneness or repeated psychophysiologic disorders.

THE DIAGNOSTIC AND PROGNOSTIC SIGNIFICANCE OF THE PAST HISTORY

As may be anticipated from the preceding section, this unraveling of the design of a patient's life into the warp and woof of his individual endowments and experiences is seldom an easy task and, in an ultimate sense, never a completed one. Nevertheless, to the physician humanely interested in his patient it is always an intriguing and revealing experience; moreover as his interviewing skills and psychiatric discernment increase, he will find that significant anamnestic information can be obtained with only a moderate outlay of time and effort. Further, the clinical indispensability of the data so acquired will become increasingly apparent, since they serve to answer questions as essential as the following: What are the patient's physical, motivational, affective and intellectual characteristics—his assets and liabilities? How rigid or pliable are his motivations, attitudes and patterns of behavior? How deep are the roots of his present neurotic aberrations, and what potentialities has he that may be utilized in fostering personal and social readaptations? Such questions are obviously of great diagnostic and prognostic import, since they seek to determine whether the patient's presenting "illness" is merely an acute reaction destined to spontaneous recovery with the abeyance of the special stresses that precipitated it, or, conversely, whether his aberrant behavior represents but a slight exacerbation of fixed and relatively unmodifiable lifetime patterns.

Herewith typical clinical examples:

CASE 12: "Combat Neurosis." A soldier suffering from physiologic exhaustion and reactions of acute anxiety as a result of overlong exposure to the physical stresses and harrowing emotional conflicts of combat would ordinarily be expected to show marked improvement if given rest, physical care and temporary surcease from danger; indeed, he should then be ready to re-enter the fray. Wartime experience, however, has adequately demonstrated that the prognosis as to the future military usefulness of the particular soldier in question would actually depend on many determinants: his group loyalties or aversions, his previous reactions to various degrees and types of deprivation, frustration and danger, his susceptibilities to recurrent anxiety and to persistent and disabling neurotic and regressive responses, and other such lifelong characteristics as can best be revealed by a study of the patient's past behavior.

CASE 13:   Acute Depressive Reaction. A 22-year-old woman was brought to the University Clinics with the history that for the preceding three months she had suffered from symptoms characteristic of a severe depression: insomnia, marked anorexia, loss of weight, despondency, fatigue, obsessive preoccupations with the possibility that somehow she had been maritally unfaithful, and recurrent ideas of suicide. The patient's account of her present illness indicated that against her family's active opposition, she had contracted a hasty but romantic marriage to a Navy petty officer after only a brief acquaintance, that he had proved to be a suspicious and hyperemotional individual, and that their marital life had been stormy and traumatic for the few weeks before he had left for a tour of sea duty. The patient was highly disturbed by his departure and became more so when, shortly afterward, a medical examination revealed that she had gonorrhea and was pregnant. Frantic letters to her husband remained unanswered and the patient, feeling abandoned and betrayed by everyone in her acute distress, reacted with the severe depression noted above.

Her past history, however, revealed that she had been a healthy, active normal child and that she had made good scholastic and social adjustments throughout her developmental years and in her university work, after which she had held responsible positions as an executive assistant. Specific inquiry disclosed only relatively minor anxiety or depressive reactions to previous frustrations and disappointments, including the death of her idolized father and the subsequent loss of her family's fortunes. In fact, she had been remarkably versatile and stable until her marriage and the concatenation of adversities previously noted had precipitated her presenting illness. The prognosis therefore seemed favorable, and treatment was directed along realistic lines.

The patient was hospitalized for protection and nursing care, the odium of venereal disease was removed insofar as possible by factual reassurances and adequate therapy, and familial reconciliations were arranged. Similarly, with the co-operation of military and Red Cross authorities, the patient's husband was located and tactfully informed of the situation. He promptly wrote her that he had not been in a position to receive her letters previously, but that he was devoted to her and was sure the child was his; moreover, he admitted that she had contracted gonorrhea from him. Within three weeks the patient had recovered her health, spirits, and self-reliance and was back at full-time work. She delivered the child without physical or psychiatric complications and continued to show normal readjustments in every sphere of behavior during a three-year follow-up.

The case just cited may be contrasted with the following:

CASE 14:   Conversion reaction in an infantile personality. An attractive, intelligent 30-year-old spinster applied for treatment with the single complaint of a slight weakness of the left arm since she had begun working in an office a month previously. On further inquiry, the patient could recollect only a few other symptoms: occasional dizzy spells, mild phobias and a tendency to social shyness. The patient agreed with her most recent physician in attributing all of these symptoms to "nervousness", although she apparently regarded the latter as a type of disease *sui generis*, "affecting her nervous system", which required only proper rest, diet and medication.

Her past history contrasted sharply with the seeming mildness of the presenting illness. She revealed feeding difficulties, night terrors and other neurotic aberrations in early childhood; marked dependence on the mother and rivalry with her younger brother; persistent enuresis until the age of thirteen; disciplinary troubles at school with frequent absenteeism for various vague illnesses; a fragmentary evolution of interests in social and recreational outlets; and diffuse phobias and inhibitions with reactions of anxiety under circumstances of even mild sexual or social stress. There had been almost no emancipation from the family in adolescence; in fact, the dependence on her mother—an aggressive, pre-emptive woman—continued so great that the patient still lived, ate, and slept with her, and could hardly bear a day's separation.

The medical history disclosed that the patient had been consulting a long succession of doctors for various complaints since childhood, and had received a vast variety of treatments, including "naturopathic" diets, chiropractic adjustments and endocrine therapy. When the patient was 16, her parents separated and sued for divorce; concurrently she developed episodes of weakness, trembling and fatigue. A thyroidectomy was performed, but the patient's symptoms showed no marked improvement until the divorce was settled and she was sure that she could live with her mother. The patient continued her attendance at various clinics, eagerly accepted new diagnoses and cooperated passively with whatever was prescribed. This practice was apparently encouraged by the mother who, by keeping the patient "ill" and ostensibly in need of constant care, was able to maintain maternal dominance. The patient was unable to work regularly; since graduation from high school at 18, she had held four jobs an average of two months, and had quit each of them to "rest" or undergo various new treatments for her long succession of illnesses.

Finally, the symptoms that occasioned her admission to the Clinics developed when she had been forced by financial needs to become a clerical worker in a large office; she had taken an instant dislike to her routine mechanical duties—which, indeed, were considerably below her intellectual capacities. At about the same time, her younger brother returned home and temporarily displaced her from her accustomed position as the center of family attention. The patient developed diffuse anxiety and the "conversion" symptoms of an arm paralysis which simultaneously denied her jealous aggressions, made work impossible and justified a return to infantile dependence. Indeed, she achieved the regressive gain of admission to a private room, doctors' and nurses' attention, and the renewed concern of her mother, who hovered over her almost constantly at the hospital. True, these advantages were obtained at the cost of certain sacrifices, such as temporary surrender of freedom and activity, but the patient's relative lack of alarm over her symptoms (la belle indifference) and her cheerfully self-prescribed course of treatment demonstrated clearly that her "disabilities" were far from unacceptable. On the contrary, as indicated by the survey of her past history, they were simply another expression of fixed patterns of infantile dependency, covertly homosexual maternal fixations and other neurotic defenses that had characterized her behavior since childhood.

The patient's rapid but unstable symptomatic "improvement" under therapy and her profession of enthusiatic but essentially spurious "insight" into her difficulties also proved instructive. As she once again formed a childishly dependent relationship to her physicians her anxiety rapidly abated; she avidly "accepted" their explanations and assurances that her paralysis had no organic basis and could be readily overcome by appropriate understanding and effort on her part. Direct suggestions combined with the prescription of arm exercises and occupational therapy readily restored complete function to the arm, and within a week the patient declared herself symptom-free. In the same way she followed the doctor's leads in discussing her excessive devotion to her mother, her jealousies of her father and her brother, her feelings of personal inferiority, and her anxieties with regard to past and current familial, sexual, social and occupational problems. She likewise volunteered data to the effect that many of her previous "illnesses" as well as her "nervous breakdowns" had been precipitated by conflicts over these problems; moreover, she admitted that any lasting recovery would entail serious attempts on her part to achieve familial emancipation, stable occupational adjustments and the development of satisfactory extrafamilial interests and social relationships.

Two weeks after her admission she was discharged, free of symptoms, professing complete "insight" and apparently intent upon sweeping changes in her ways of living. And yet, the poor prognosis indicated by her past performances was entirely justified by a follow-up study of her case two years later. At that time it was learned that two days after her discharge from the hospital, the patient had "accidentally" slipped down a short flight of stairs at the first place she applied for a position and immediately had developed back pains and "weakness of the legs". Neurologists and orthopedic physicians who were called into consultation could find no evidence of physical injury; nevertheless, the patient spent the next month once again recuperating under her mother's tender care. At the end of this period, anorexia and other mild but presistent organic dysfunctions reappeared and the patient quickly relapsed into her accustomed rounds of chiropractors, naturopaths, and other assorted "healers" and "counsellors".

As may be seen from these brief examples, the immediate clinical diagnosis must be supplemented with—and is in an important sense actually dependent upon—a survey of the total personality as determined by an organized and evaluative study of the patient's life patterns. In the first case cited the usual nosologic labels of "reactive depression," "melancholia," or "agitated tension state" would indicate only the leading features of the patient's current reactions, but would give insufficient indication that she was a relatively able, mature and competent individual who had succumbed to a combination of unusually severe emotional stresses. In the last case, neither the diagnosis of "conversion reaction, mild" with reference to the patient's presenting arm symptoms, nor her rapid "recovery" under simple treatment would have revealed the fact, apparent mainly from a careful evaluation of her past history, that she was a dependent, uneman- cipated, immature individual with almost intractable tendencies toward neurotic and regressive reactions under circumstances which seemed to threaten, however remotely, her needs for infantile security. True, her response to brief forms of therapy in the Clinics indicated a certain plastic- ity in her reactions, but her symptomatic "recovery" was merely a function of her temporary desire to seek the physician's approval and protection, and thus was in itself merely a part of her neurosis; certainly, when her dependent needs once again were elicited by her mother, her former pat- terns of aberrant adaptation reappeared unchanged.

Parenthetically, in the last case, as in many others, the past history likewise served the important function of revealing a character neurosis in the patient's mother that complemented the patient's own and thus made the prospects of recovery in either case even more remote. But even if it had been possible to separate the two, work intensively with the patient to establish operationally effective rather than merely verbal insight, and then give her every advantage and guidance in various spheres of adaptation, in view of her past history of twenty-eight years of neurotic ways of living— however mild their clinical manifestations—there would still remain a con- siderable doubt as to whether she could be fundamentally changed by any form of therapy. As will be seen in later clinical sections, the eventual out- come of any given case actually depends on a multiplicity of interrelated factors, not all of which are under either the patient's or the physician's con- trol. However, as may now be evident, an objective examination of the pa- tient's anamnesis can furnish immediate and important leads not only as to diagnosis, but also as to prognosis and therapy.

REFERENCES

1. Grinker, R. R., Sr., Weible, Beatrice and Drye, R. C.: *The Borderline Syndrome*. New York, Basic Books, 1968.
2. Menninger, K. A.: *A Manual for Psychiatric Case Study*. New York, Grune & Stratton, 1952.
3. Ripley, H. S.: The psychiatric interview. *In* Freedman, A. M. and Kaplan, H. (Eds.): *Comprehensive Textbook of Psychiatry*. Baltimore, Williams & Williams, 1967.
4. Ruesch, J. and Bateson, G.: *Communication, the Social Matrix of Psychiatry*. New York, W. W. Norton, 1959.
5. Whitehorn, J. C.: Guide to interviewing. *Arch. Neurol. & Psychiat.* 52:197, 1944.

Chapter 3

TECHNIQUES OF THE PSYCHIATRIC EXAMINATION

In previous sections we have discussed the objectives, content and significance of the psychiatric history; there remain to be considered, however, the various methods by which the anamnestic examination may best be conducted. These techniques, like those employed in psychotherapy, have often been referred to as an "intuitive art"—and this is true to the extent that intuition in psychiatry, as elsewhere, means mainly depth and immediacy of understanding derived from unverbalized knowledge through experience, and *art* in this context implies sensitivity and finesse in human relationships. The physician's facility in sensing and responding to his patients' verbal and non-verbal communications generally increases along with his therapeutic skill; nevertheless, preliminary training in dynamic psychiatry serves to give direction and speed to this progress. Since the first psychiatric interview is not only important from a diagnostic standpoint but also greatly influences all future relationships between the physician and patient, it is imperative that methods be employed that will serve diagnostic and therapeutic purposes to the best advantage. The practices outlined below, properly modified to suit the individual case, will be found useful.

PRELIMINARY CONSIDERATIONS

Some patients are still obviously hesitant about consulting a psychiatrist because of the "stigma" attached to mental illness (e.g., sometimes a husband or wife wishes to obtain psychiatric consultation without the spouse knowing about it), unsureness about the need for or wisdom of such action and covert or overt desires to retain cherished patterns of conduct. On initial contact, therefore, the receptionist or nurse should be trained to assure the prospective patient by a quiet, friendly greeting and a warm but discreet manner—and verbally in some instances—that his attendance will be completely voluntary, and that his identity and all other data will be kept confidential. Except when circumstances necessitate a visit to the home or the hospital bedside, the psychiatric interview is best held in the therapist's private office. Here a proper physical setting is helpful: modest, home-like furnishings, restful pictures on the wall, an easy chair for the patient, facilities for smoking, an anteroom for resting or primping after an interview—

all these foster a feeling of ease and security in anxious or sensitive patients. Incidentally, a photograph of the physician's wife and children on his desk often serves silently but well in forestalling or controlling unrealistic or undesirable deviations of transference.

Privacy in the Interview

Whatever the patient's conscious pretexts for the visit, it must be remembered that he comes to the therapist because of his needs for individualized attention, and that during the course of the interview he may wish to impart highly confidential information about himself or others. When it appears likely that the patient may later regret or resent an excessive burst of confidence, this tendency may be temporarily checked; however, in most cases a reasonable degree of anamnestic catharsis may be encouraged if it relieves the patient, furnishes the examiner with diagnostic information, and aids in developing rapport. The initial interchanges, therefore, should be conducted as privately as a confessional, and whenever possible outsiders should be excluded. When the patient is accompanied by the fond mother, the complaining or compliant spouse, or the helpful but curious neighbor, the companion should be requested to wait until the patient is interviewed. When a companion is consulted first, the patient may assume the role of a martyr who is misunderstood and unjustly accused, regard the psychiatrist as a magistrate, and spend the time remaining for him in answering supposed allegations or raising counter-charges to justify his conduct. Only after the patient is examined should other informants be seen and, except for emergencies, even then only with the patient's expressed permission and in his presence. Following these guidelines avoids all semblance of an inquisition; the patient feels that he alone is the special object of the physician's care. With frankly psychotic patients these rules have less immediate force; sometimes it is necessary to see the informants first and separately. However, even in such cases, the physician may be surprised to learn, perhaps long afterward, how important his first contacts with agitated or withdrawn patients may have been, or that requesting the patient's permission to see other informants, even as a seeming formality, may have dispelled some doubts about and fostered confidence in the physician. In the case of epileptic, hyperemotional, delirious or markedly delusional patients it is not only permissible, but may be advisable to have a third person present throughout the interview.

Case Notes

Although there are a number of reasons against recording the patient's history in his presence, or even taking notes during the psychiatric interview, with few exceptions the examiner should handle this matter in the way in which he and the patient are most comfortable. Some patients appreciate the full, concentrated attention of the examiner and may speak more spontaneously and freely when remarks are not being recorded. Further, if the examiner is distracted by note-taking he may fail to observe many meaningful nunances in the patient's behavior; in any case short, accurate summaries can be written after the patient has left. Conversely, some patients may regard the interviewer's unobtrusive recording as evidence of thoroughness and professional interest.

With every patient, the physician should discuss the matter of professional records with frankness and complete honesty. When the physician mentions that he is taking notes or making short summaries in order to record certain bits of information which he will use solely to maintain continuity and to study, usually the patient not only appreciates the physician's candor, but also wishes him to proceed in his accustomed, professional way. Thus the patient should be informed about the written record and the necessity for keeping it; as one incentive, some insurance companies will not provide third-party payments unless a written record is kept. But in all cases, the physician should inform the patient that his record and all correspondence dealing with him will not contain any information of a highly confidential or potentially embarrassing nature, which might—even if subpoenaed—be used against him. However, referring briefly to notes for a few minutes *prior to seeing the patient* rather than in his presence refreshes the physician's memory, and reassures the patient that his therapist remembers the details of his case from session to session.

Attitudes toward Previous Therapists

While discussing his medical history, the patient may begin to inveigh against former physicians for "mistakes" in diagnosis, ineffectual treatments and "needless" operations, just as he may blame former psychotherapists for "misleading" advice which increased his difficulties. Under such circumstances the inexperienced interviewer, flattered by the patient's implied or overtly complimentary comparisons, may be inclined either to listen sympathetically to these criticisms, or at best maintain a professionally aloof or strictly "neutral" attitude. Either of these postures is generally inadvisable, since even on the relatively rare occasions when the criticisms are deserved, they are expressed by the patient with the unconscious purpose of maneuvering the interviewer into agreeing, openly or tacitly, that professional people have made serious errors in diagnosis and therapy and that therefore "they"—and this now includes the examiner—may also do so in the future. Generally, such criticisms of past "mishandling" are really a covert attack on the present interviewer; in fact, if this type of defensive aggressivity on the patient's part continues unrecognized and unchallenged, it will almost inevitably be turned into increasing distrust of, and diminishing cooperation with, the current therapist, who will ultimately be maligned in his turn. Good technique as well as good ethics demands that, instead of joining in his rancor, adequate explanations be given the patient to the effect that the advice and treatment he may have received from previous physicians might indeed have been indicated at the time. A general formula for such reassurances, whenever applicable, may run as follows:

> "I have no personal knowledge of the doctors or other therapists you consulted, and I certainly cannot make any judgment about the advice and treatment which they gave you and which they considered necessary. If you wish, I will write or consult them about their findings and the reasons for and the results of their treatment. In any case, the important thing for us to consider is your present condition and what can be done about it from now on."

BEGINNING THE INTERVIEW

After a simple, friendly introductory greeting the interviewer should invite the patient to "Tell me what is troubling you." The development of the interview is then contingent upon the patient's responsive gambit. Sometimes a patient who has been referred by another physician assumes that the interviewer is thoroughly familiar with "his case." When this happens it is best for the interviewer to tell the patient simply that he was given a few facts by the referring physician but that they are not sufficient, and that it is best for the patient to relate his history as he wishes. On occasion, a patient may become speechless after entering the office; when this occurs, the interviewer should permit the patient to be quiet for a few minutes and then indicate tactfully that he is aware that it may be difficult to begin talking immediately, but that the patient should attempt to do so and just start anywhere he or she wishes. Understanding the patient's reticence and possible embarrassment and quietly conveying that understanding often suffices to avert an impasse.

If as is frequent, the patient begins hesitantly asking advice about occupational, sexual, or social difficulties, this initial lead may be followed, although the interviewer should be aware that in all probability the problems the patient approaches first are not necessarily the most pathogenic ones, and that a much fuller survey of his maladjustments will have to be made. On the other hand, an occasional patient may begin to pour out a stream of confessions too freely; in such instances the interviewer should be aware that this, in itself, may be indicative of poor control and should use the first opportunity to protect the patient by tactful inquiries designed to develop the history in a more systematic fashion.

A number of patients begin the interview with a listing of somatic complaints and symptoms, embellished with an account of previous diagnoses, operations, and treatments. When this occurs, the interviewer will generally find that it is best to listen to the patient's account of his illness with manifest care. Initial suspiciousness, extreme defenseness, or even truculence is often lulled by a sympathetic hearing, while at the same time the physician may obtain valuable information about the patient's attitudes and defense mechanisms, as well as the onset, duration, and presence of symptomatic expressions of anxiety, depression, psychophysiologic illnesses, etc. Indeed, if the patient has a strongly defensive need to believe that he is physically ill, or if he has not had an adequate medical examination recently, it may be advisable to defer extensive psychiatric history-taking until he has had a thorough medical check-up and the reports of laboratory or other special diagnostic studies have been obtained. The patient may welcome a direct physical examination, or consider the psychiatrist's referral to an internist for a more thorough medical work-up as evidence of professional competence.

APPROACH TO PSYCHIATRIC DATA

Here, another impasse may occur which requires further skillful handling. Some patients may seize upon such referrals to assert that all their physical and behavioral difficulties have an organic basis which would indeed be discovered if only further examinations were undertaken to find the hereditary, toxic, or other cause of their "nervousness." Occasionally, a patient may admit that he has serious problems in living and may even be "neurotic," but yet refuse to see the relevance of dissatisfactions, problems, and emotional disturbances to his physical complaints, let alone explore the actual maladjustments and conflicts which might have an etiologic bearing on his difficulties. In such circumstances, initial insight on the patient's part may be encouraged by simple clarifications which avoid technical terms but which nevertheless make clear the everyday relationships between life stresses and both emotional and physical disturbances. For example, a patient who is subject to physical manifestations of anxiety attacks, yet who cannot understand why his symptoms do not constitute evidence that he has heart disease, may be given an explanation such as the following:

> "All of us have been extremely frightened at one time or another by a near collision or the danger of a wreck. As human beings, we react emotionally

and physically to such threats of danger and develop certain symptoms such as a fast heart, shortness of breath, a lump in the throat, a tightness in the chest, a cold sweat, and feelings of trembling or weakness. When this occurs and when we know that it is related to obvious danger, we call it a 'nervous reaction.' However, sometimes the fear persists so that one becomes tense when he is in an automobile, hears the sounds of speeding vehicles or even approaches a certain intersection where he almost had an accident. In these circumstances, a person tends to feel vaguely uneasy and may have a return of severe symptoms without knowing why. In fact, even if he didn't know he was afraid, let alone what he was afraid of, his heart might keep pounding or his knees feel weak and trembly until he remembered that, although he had once been badly scared by something, there was nothing to be frightened about anymore. The main difference between such a situation and the spells of palpitations and faintness which trouble you now is that you have not yet figured out their cause. Perhaps you and I can find out what hidden fears still make you tense or apprehensive every day, and so bring on the 'nervous symptoms' you describe."

Of course, the nature, content, and phrasing of such explanations must be adapted to the intelligence and receptivity of the patient, and must be specifically designed to apply to his presenting complaints. The affective setting of various dysfunctions such as gastrointestinal disturbances, enuresis, or attacks of "dizziness and faintness" can be approached by illustrations that are meaningful to the specific patient in terms of his own conscious experiences. For example, the neurotic background in a case of functional vomiting may be approached in the following vein:

"As you see (summarize briefly the negative physical diagnostic findings and emphasize that the patient has had a thorough medical work-up), we can both be relieved that there is no evidence of serious physical illness. But all of us can understand, from personal experience, that even a physically healthy organ can function abnormally when a person is emotionally disturbed by serious problems. For instance, all of us know that perfectly strong, healthy men may become weak and faint at the sight of blood, or, that another person may become nauseated and vomit when he is feeling ashamed, afraid, disgusted, or angry. Now, let's examine the kind of feelings that seem to bring on your symptoms."

The conflictual origin of reactions such as phobias, obsessions, or compulsions can be approached by citing some childhood experience with which almost everyone can identify. A useful example is the following:

"Suppose a two- or three-year-old child is left alone in a house at dusk. He wanders into a dark room and sees a high, white object move threateningly in a corner; he becomes terrified and runs away; later, when he tries to tell his parents about this experience he's not understood or he's laughed at. But the child may begin to be afraid of the dark, of large moving objects, or perhaps even of the color white; for example, he may grow to dislike white clothes, or be unable to sleep on white sheets. He may develop little habits of tiptoeing past doors, wetting the bed, or of grabbing people's hands when he enters a room. Soon, the parents guess what has happened, talk to him about it, take him back to the dark room where he was frightened and show him that all he saw were familiar and harmless white curtains blowing about. But if they don't do that, the child, even though he no longer clearly remembers his original experience, may continue to have all sorts of unusual fears and protective habits in later life. You wouldn't call him 'physically sick,' nor would you call him either 'unintelligent' or 'insane.' He's just frightened of things that he never came to understand or control. I think that you can begin to see that there's no reason to think of yourself in terms of illness, or be ashamed because you have the fears or habits you came to see me about. It is a question of tracing them to happenings in the past that may have started them off—and then getting you to see that the fears and habits are perhaps no longer necessary."

Such examples and explanations, it should be reemphasized, must be suited in language, content, complexity of concept, and directness of application to the individual patient; if not, these or other stock stories, diagrams, or formulas often defeat their own purpose. Certain additional cautions may be specifically mentioned:

Impersonality in Illustration. Never cite the actual history of another patient; even an anonymous account would not only violate medical ethics but also diminish the patient's trust in the completely inviolate nature of the anamnestic material he himself might give you.

Generality. All explanations should be phrased hypothetically, or else the patient, instead of being stimulated to examine his own past and present problems, may passively accept the explanation as an "interpretation" of his own case and let the matter rest there. It is best to present illustrations and generalizations as common experiences which, at least to some degree in fantasy or in fact, are applicable to all of humanity. When a patient begins to realize that his fears and behaviors, which he may regard as highly abnormal, differ primarily only in degree from the fears and behaviors of all mankind, he will not only begin to talk about them more openly but also come to look upon himself as not being an absolutely unusual individual. His level of self-esteem then increases, often permitting him to relinquish some of his neurotic defenses.

Precautions against Overreaction. Anxiety-cathected material should not be approached too precipitately, since the patient may become defensive and resentful, react by breaking off the therapeutic contact, or even develop states of depression and panic with suicidal tendencies. The following case is a pertinent example:

CASE 15: Personality pattern disturbance with suicidal reactions to injudicious interpretations. A woman with a highly moralistic upbringing developed anxiety attacks, obsessive fears of germs, and a severe hand-washing compulsion after her husband failed in business and forced her to move their family of five children to a squalid dwelling among slum surroundings. She consulted various physicians who, ignoring the manifestly neurotic features of her illness, diagnosed "thyroid trouble" or heart disease as the basis of her palpitations, tremors, and elevated metabolic rate. However, the patient showed little improvement from medications, refused a thyroidectomy recommended by one physician, and was finally referred to a therapist who, without special training in the field, claimed to practice "psychoanalysis." After only two initial interviews she was told by him that he knew exactly what was wrong with her: she hated her husband and children, wanted to kill them, and therefore, like Lady Macbeth, kept washing their blood off her hands. The patient, angry and incredulous, broke off the "treatment," but could not shake off the memory of the awful accusation. Her anxieties, obsessions and self-accusatory ruminations increased and one day, in a state of melancholic agitation, she attempted to poison two of the younger children and herself "to save the family from insanity." Symbolically and fortunately, she used only an overdose of a minor tranquilizer previously prescribed by one of her physicians, and all three patients responded quickly to treatment soon after hospitalization. Fortunately, too. subsequent therapy, properly graduated over a period of a year and combined with marital and social readjustments, greatly alleviated the patient's neurosis. This case serves to illustrate how a highly injudicious pseudoanalytic "interpretation"—though containing some truth in a symbolic sense—may shatter a patient's brittle but essential defenses and precipitate reactions of anxiety and depression which may have grave consequences.

Flight to the Remote. Every effort should be made to keep the information being gathered from the patient as closely related to current realities as possible. When this is not done, many patients—in preference to facing their hard problems in the here and now—inveigle the inexperienced examiner into listening to endless recollections about remote, dimly remembered, and inevitably misinterpreted past experiences. This may be permitted for a time, but eventually the patient must be brought back to his current behavior—the only reality, after all, that can be changed by the physician's or the patient's efforts. When, therefore, sufficient rapport and initial insight have been established, the necessary transition may be made by a statement such as the following:

"A person's early experience may make him specially sensitive to disappointments or failures, and he can continue to be deeply troubled, even by minor aggravations, the rest of his life without realizing how seriously his peace of mind and his health are affected. But then, it's very important to know what might be upsetting you *now*. Generally, if we face it frankly, it

turns out to be not too mysterious: it may be family disagreements, sexual difficulties, an unsatisfactory social life, financial troubles, overwork or other
circumstances to which one has become sensitive. Please tell me about your
daily life, what you do, what you feel, and what troubles you."

Despite the seeming superficiality and triteness of such verbal maneuvers, they have a number of advantages which have been confirmed by
experience. Obviously, they focus attention on the present; more subtly,
they also lull the patient's anxieties and diminish his defensiveness by
assuring him (a) that the interviewer is understanding and sympathetic, (b)
that the interviewer is experienced and realistic, and (c) that anxiety-ridden
topics such as sexual and familial difficulties or social maladjustments may
be discussed as objectively as financial difficulties, "overwork," or current
business troubles. Of course, even if the patient avidly seizes on the latter
as a topic of first choice, his material on that score will at least deal with
current stresses, and thus lead to discussions of insecurity or competitiveness at work, hostilities to superiors, feelings of inadequacy, and so on.
Once so started, examiner and patient may proceed to explore more deeply
guarded material in other spheres of living which is directly related to the
patient's current maladjustments.

DEVELOPMENT OF THE PSYCHIATRIC HISTORY

To obtain a meaningful account of the patient's life history and the stresses
and problems which now ensue, the interviewer should aim to develop a
coherent, congruent human story. True, the interviewer is obliged to obtain
data, say, about the "family history," since it may reveal events and forces
which bear on the patient's current situation as well as his growth and
development. However, the interviewer should not unduly interrupt the
patient's spontaneous communications because of a compulsive need to be
"thorough and complete." Stereotyped questions and awkward transitions
lead the patient to think that the physician is "merely following a form"
and thus diminish rapport as well as disrupt coherence. Throughout the
examination such reactions can be prevented by applying a principle fundamental to all interviewing techniques—that of *motivational relativity*. This
principle can be elaborated more explicitly as follows:
    Conduct the interview so that the patient accepts each succeeding step
as being relevant to his personal interests and, in all probability, beneficial
to him. Thought and skill should be used in arranging the interview so that
the patient not only feels but also begins to realize that it is to his advantage to offer information about his past and familial histories, and that the
interviewer seeks such material only for the patient's sake. An easy transi-

tion between the patient's account of his present illness and significant aspects of his past experiences and early neurotic reactions may take the following simple form:

> "You can see now (after a brief summary of the current setting of his presenting complaints) that you are a rather high-strung and sensitive person. Some people develop such characteristics quite early in life; in fact, even in childhood. Can you remember being shy and sensitive when you were a child, too? (and, to lead into a family history) Was that characteristic of others in your family?"

Obviously, inquiries of this type indicate the examiner's acceptance rather than condemnation of the patient's personality difficulties and disclose his desire to trace their roots in a thorough and helpful manner. Moreover, this technique prepares the patient to accept more specific questions about both his early formative reactions and current difficulties as presented in Chapter 2.

Semantic Acceptability

It is necessary to emphasize another principle adhered to in all the examples thus far quoted—a principle that makes the questions appear stilted when read, yet renders them effective when asked with proper warmth and intonation in personal contact. This principle is: *In the language of the psychiatric interview, employ terms which, in the patient's meaning-system, are not charged with any hint of disapproval or opprobrium.*

Many patients who, for example, may readily accept the statement that they are "high-strung", "emotionally hypersensitive", or "overmeticulous" deeply resent any hints that they now or ever have been "irritable", "unstable" or "compulsive". The interviewer, therefore, must be exceedingly careful about the use of terms which the patient may interpret as condemnatory of himself or, when taking his past history, of various members of his family.

Family History

To maintain coherence, certain simple techniques for making transitions to various portions of the history can be employed. Thus, in investigating the patient's early relationships it is smooth and simple to invite him to describe those of his relatives as well as of friends, teachers, or others, who appear to have played major roles in his life. When his descriptions indicate that his experiences with some particular persons were especially significant, the patient may be asked whether that person, too, was "overly sensitive," or tended to become "emotionally upset," as an introduction to more specific questioning. His replies on this score are generally most significant with regard to parents, siblings, and spouse, although, as indicated under "Mental Status" (Chapter 4), this usually reveals as much or more about the patient's own attitudes toward the person in question than it does about the latter's "actual" characteristics, past or present.

Sexual History

This should be approached tactfully, objectively, and helpfully. With women, an acceptable starting point is the menstrual history, which provides an easy transition to obtaining information about early sexual fantasies, memories, erotic play and masturbation; sexual experiences and guilts; disturbances of orgasm; physical and emotional reactions to pregnancy; and current sexual activities and satisfactions or dissatisfactions. With men, the subject may be opened by an initial, routine inquiry into the frequency and adequacy of erections and intercourse, leading to supplementary accounts of previous erotic experiences, emotional reactions, and fantasies. Often, with both men and women, inquiring about how and when they first learned about sexual activity is a simple initial way to obtain the sexual history.

Inquiries about deviant sexual practices may sometimes be approached when the interviewer senses that the patient's immediate confidences on this score will be helpful rather than disturbing. With the degree of frankness about sexuality that is part of our contemporary scene, many patients wish to talk about their sexual activities openly, and expect to be asked about them. Generally, however, a detailed discussion of various sexual activities is more meaningful when it is placed in its proper context, i.e., when the interviewer can discern what the sexual activities mean to the patient and how they influence his interpersonal relationships.

REFERENCES

1. Blum, R. H.: *The Management of the Doctor-Patient Relationship.* New York, McGraw-Hill, 1960.
2. Deutsch, F. and Murphy, W. F.: *The Clinical Interview.* New York, International Universities Press, 1955.
3. Hoch, P. H.: *Differential Diagnosis in Clinical Psychiatry.* New York, Science House, 1973.
4. Mayer-Gross, W., Slater, E., and Roth, M: *Clinical Psychiatry.* Baltimore, Williams and Wilkins, 1955.
5. Menninger, K.: *A Manual for Psychiatric Case Study.* New York, Grune & Stratton, 1952.
6. Redlich, F. C. and Freedman, D. X.: *Theory and Practice of Psychiatry.* New York, Basic Books, Inc., 1966.

Chapter 4

CURRENT BEHAVIORAL OR "MENTAL STATUS" EXAMINATION

As has been seen, the "past psychiatric history" is an integration of reports, often from a number of sources, about the patient's characteristic patterns of behavior, and the "present illness" is an account of the disturbances that resulted from various stresses and conflicts. But since all such accounts are necessarily colored and distorted by each informant's own biases and attitudes, it is necessary to evaluate all anamnestic information in the light of the informant's observed behavior. The direct scrutiny of the patient leads to an evaluation of his "mental status" and is of paramount diagnostic importance.

PARALLELISM OF DIRECT PSYCHIATRIC EXAMINATION AND MEDICAL DIAGNOSIS

The psychiatric appraisal of a patient's "mental status" has sometimes been misinterpreted as analogous to "mind reading"—a series of subjective judgments about "mental aberrations." But in actuality it is a relatively objective procedure, comparable in many respects to the physical examination employed in medical diagnosis. To illustrate: The cardiologist is first interested in the patient's present illness, e.g., the nature and intensity of recent symptoms of cardiac decompensation (dyspnea, chest pain, edema) and their relationships to special stresses such as overexertion or exposure to high altitudes. Next, the cardiologist examines the possible etiologic background of such symptoms in the past history: the susceptibilities of the patient's family to heart disease (hereditary factors), the occurrence of congenital abnormalities or of cardiac traumata at birth, the pathogenic effects of illnesses such as rheumatic fever during childhood and later life, and the nature of the morbid influences that finally precipitated the "present illness." With this anamnestic material at hand, he next proceeds to examine the patient's cardiovascular functions by inspection, palpation, auscultation, and percussion, and more indirectly by X-ray, electrocardiography, and other technical means. Having completed various observations of the patient's cardiovascular functions under "resting" conditions, he may then direct his patient to perform specially designed exercises in order to observe the performance of his cardiovascular system under known and standardized stresses.

So also, the psychiatric anamnesis first records the nature and intensity of the complaints and symptoms constituting the "presenting illness," with particular reference to the possible etiology of specific dysfunctions and their alleviation or exacerbation under various circumstances. During the process of history-taking, the interviewer also observes the patient's "spontaneous" behavior and finally proceeds, whenever indicated, to study his responses to various questionnaires or performance tests, reactions to drugs, or changes under hypnosis. Although total behavior is complex, it may still be studied objectively, analyzed as to structure and function, and interpreted in diagnostically and pragmatically meaningful terms.

ORGANIZATION OF THE DATA

During the history-taking the patient's manner and speech, his verbal associations and evasions, his attitudes toward the physician, his emotional reactions, and many other phenomena will, when carefully noted and interpreted, reveal much about his conative, intellectual, and affective characteristics. To promote clarity of observation and organization, these phenomena may be grouped as follows:

General Appearance

Appropriate, agitated, exhibitionistic, or withdrawn.

Dress: Tasteful, excessively neat, overmodest, or garish, sloppy, in disarray.

Bearing: Relaxed, tense, defiant, martyred, overburdened, crushed.

Facial Expression: Cheerful, animated, impassive, vacuous, dazed, harassed, anxious, melancholic, distorted.

Stream of Talk

Fluency, ease of expression, accent, clarity, rapidity, pressure, hesitancies, blocking, repetitiousness, stuttering, transient aphasias. Severe and persistent deviations from normal such as verbigeration (repetition of words), echolalia (automatic repetition of the examiner's words), or neologisms (nonsense words) are pathognomonic of psychotic thought processes.

Motor Activity

Idiosyncracies of posture and motion (including tics and mannerisms); push of activity, ranging from general restlessness to slowness and retardation. Ataxia, drooling or Parkinson-like tremors may indicate drug intake. Grossly psychotic disturbances such as fixed immobility, stereotypies, bizarre exhibitionism, delusional behavior or soiling can be expected only in delirious or psychotic patients.

Estimation of Intellectual Capacities

Intellectual functions are compounded of many diverse perceptive, mnemonic, integrative, abstractive, and operational abilities. Despite the interplay of these functions, a fair estimate of the patient's general capacities may be made on the basis of the following criteria:

Wealth of General Information: This indicates previous and current interests and activities, preservation of memory, and availability of rapid recall.

General Education, Cultural Level, and Special Talents: Completing nine or more years in a public school generally indicates that the patient possessed at least low normal intelligence; if he graduated from high school with reasonable standards, his general abilities were at one time at least within normal range. Highly specialized attainments, however, may be an uncertain index of general intelligence; e.g., a memory expert, a lightning calculator, a master chess player, or a skillful craftsman may or may not have other capacities commensurate with his limited superiorities in memory, arithmetic, field-perception, or special motor skills. On the other hand, broader occupational, social, cultural, and artistic attainments correlate well with higher levels of general intelligence.

Communication: Since symbolization, idea-integration and verbalization combine some of the most complex cerebral functions, the patient's use of language is usually an excellent index of his general intellectual capacities (cf. sections on intelligence tests and aphasia in Chapter 6). From a clinical standpoint, his spoken or written productions may be appraised as follows:

Vocabulary. The mere *size* of a person's vocabulary is not an infallible index of his general intelligence, since it may be padded with occupational and technical terms learned merely by rote or words not appropriately understood or used. On the other hand, new words are continually acquired by persons who excel in certain higher intellectual capacities, with the result that their vocabularies become correspondingly rich in the following categories:

Specific names of things. To a very young child the simple term "stick" is an adequate name for a cane, a slide rule, a toy soldier or a jib boom; later, as finer perceptions develop, his differential vocabulary increases.

Qualifications of objects. Coincident with development, the objects themselves are further qualified from the simple "short" or "thick" cane to the more complexly "rigged" jib boom or the "logarithmically graduated" slide rule.

Spatial translation of objects. Concepts of change, motion, or growth necessitate another category of words ranging from the child's simple "fall" or "push" to the theoretical scientist's transformations of space, mass, and time.

Capacity for abstraction. Even naming objects involves some taxonomic capacities; but higher degrees of generalization, such as concepts relative to broader category formations, physical laws, mathematical equations, or social principles, require another repertoire of terms which indicates the patient's facility in these intellectual functions. As simple examples, a child learns to make a donation in school or church long before he understands the concept "charity." Or a mental retardate can learn slowly and specifically that $4 \times 4 = 16$—representing a relatively low degree of abstractive capacity—yet never be able to grasp the *principle* of multiplication.

Richness of ideation. The patient's language is assembled into phrases, clauses and sentences which, by their structure, logical consistency, wealth of imagery, and progression may range from monosyllabic grunts to scholarly discourses.

Organic disturbances of speech function may range from the covert to the obvious. Thus, aphasic lacunae in speech after a cerebral injury may easily be covered—after a hardly detectable hesitation—by the substitution of another word or phrase, or they may result in completely blocked communication (see below). Verbal substitutions in organic deficiencies accompanying brain tumors, paresis or Alzheimer's disease may take the form of inept humor ("witzelsucht") or pointlessly scatologic, profane expressions. In Korsakoff's syndrome, inconsistent and often impossible fabrications are uncritically offered as facts.

Factors in intelligence. The criteria for estimating intellectual functions are mainly useful for evaluating the patient's spontaneous productions during the clinical interview. Furthermore, the impressions gained from the interview can be translated roughly into the more specific terms used in various types of psychologic analysis. In fact, with increasing experience the clinician will acquire a justifiable confidence in his ability to estimate not only his patient's basic intellectual capacities, but also the nature and extent of the impairments in various intellectual functions.

Brief Supplementary Tests

When the patient's performance is analyzed according to the above criteria during the interview, supplementary "tests" of memory, recall, mathematical ability and abstraction may be unnecessary. Moreover, when used tactlessly, these tests may arouse the patient's suspicions and resentments. If the examiner wishes to confirm his initial impression of borderline intellectual deficiency, organic deterioration, or other such deviations, it is sometimes better to refer the patient for psychological testing rather than impair the rapport and continuity of the psychiatric interview by asking isolated "test" questions. However, as the interviewer gains experience in conducting the examination, he learns that most patients accept routine questions (e.g., about memory and calculations) as part of the complete examination and as evidence of professional thoroughness, especially after rapport has been established and at a time when it does not disrupt continuity or interfere with spontaneous expression. When it is apparent early in the interview that the patient's intellectual functions are impaired, the examiner should proceed to conduct simple tests with which to evaluate the remainder of the personal history. Finding out, for example, that a patient's memory is impaired alerts the examiner to the necessity of structuring the interview and guiding the patient by directed inquiries.

A patient's reactions to a simple mental status examination are of considerable diagnostic and prognostic importance. The patient's reluctance to cooperate or his petulance and irritability about being asked simple questions betrays his characterologic difficulties and may be evidence in itself of neurotic sensitivity or of diminished self-esteem.

Whether the patient will react with resentment and irritation to the formal mental examination depends primarily on the way it is presented to him and its timing. When an interviewer feels secure, is not anxious, and has already conveyed by his general manner his respect for the patient, even a mathematician will not object to being asked to do serial sevens. The importance of the formal mental status examination is illustrated by the following case:

CASE 16. A 32-year-old author, the wife of a college professor, sought psychiatric help because she had been extremely agitated and had serious difficulty sleeping for two weeks. While discussing her current marital problems, she talked feverishly and incessantly, made frequent references to heroines in novels, and used many literary expressions. The examiner had difficulty evaluating her history and the severity of her emotional distress until she was asked to interpret the proverb, "People who live in glass houses shouldn't throw stones." She stopped for a moment as if dazed and then replied: "My husband is like a stone—a stone is a rock—Gibraltar is a rock." Further examination indicated that her frequent literary references were evidence of loosening of associations and were not literary symbolisms. Although she denied that she had had psychiatric treatment in the past, her mother told that she had been hospitalized at the age of 18 for schizophrenia.

The patient had responded fairly accurately on a few simple tests of memory and ability to calculate but appeared distracted. Then, when her capacity for abstraction was tested, she revealed the concreteness and personalization indicative of a schizophrenic thought disorder. The results of the brief mental status examination enabled the somewhat baffled interviewer to arrive at the correct diagnosis quickly.

In interview techniques, especially those designed for screening and evaluation of intellectual functions, some of the following may be employed as tests of minimal normal performance.

Intellectual Functions

Flow of Ideation: Write a nine-word sentence; time limit, 15 seconds. Name 28 objects at random; time limit, one minute.

Reading : Read a fifty-word paragraph of ordinary narrative text in 35 seconds.

Immediate Configurative Recall: Six digits given at intervals of a second and repeated by the subject; four digits recalled in reverse order.

Progressive Subtraction: Subtract 7 from 100, then from 93 and continue as rapidly as possible. Note impairment in speed, uncorrected errors and confusions.

Conceptual Differentiations: Difference between a lie and a mistake. Or (at a lower level) between a fly and a butterfly.

Speech Recall and Reproduction: Repetition of the traditional "Around the rugged rock the ragged rascal ran." Stumbling, unclear enunciation and the omission or telescoping of words may indicate aphasic disturbances and impairments of phonetic control that occur in the organic dementias, particularly paresis.

The Sensorium

Memory: This function involves (a) the apperception, (b) the organized retention, and (c) the ready recall of visual, auditory, tactile, and other configurations of experience. Especially vivid recollections of particularly meaningful "events" should be noted, but often such accounts, especially if referred to very early life, represent *screen memories*, i.e., retrospectively falsified fantasies and symbolic distortions of what actually occurred. As we have seen, such screen memories may be significant of repressed wishes related to the patient's current behavior--in this sense, they are significant; however, the events described should not be regarded as historical fact. Conversely, *hysterical amnesias* may blot out whole segments of experience; such amnesias, unlike those caused by cerebral injury, are related to adaptational stresses, are usually selective and incomplete, and may be partially or wholly circumvented by skillful inquiry as well as by hypnosis, the administration of drugs or other methods. The patchy amnesias of chronic cerebral disease are usually characterized by a retention of old memories and a loss of recent ones: grandfather in his dotage may forget where he put his glasses but can remember in shining detail his every experience while serving in World War I.

Orientation

This concerns time, place, and interpersonal relationships as usually discerned in the mental status.

Acute disorders of orientation in all spheres occur in various toxic states and are sometimes accompanied—as in alcoholic delirium tremens— by kaleidoscopic illusions, hallucinations, and fear reactions that can reach panic proportions. Other drugs, however, such as marijuana or some of the opium derivatives, produce disorientation, somnolence and stupor from which the subject can be only temporarily roused.

Time: Of the three spheres of orientation, the sense of time is the one which is disturbed most frequently in patients with mental disorders. But there is tremendous individual variation in both the "normal" sense of the passage of time and awareness of the exact time. Punctuality and attentiveness to time are characteristics of our dominant middle-class society, but are not present to the same degree in various subcultural groups even in the United States. Moreover, every person has his own tempo of optimal activity which he can more or less consciously measure against solar time. Thus, many persons can wake spontaneously at 5:00 a.m. to keep an anticipated early morning golf date, but need an insistent alarm to rouse them at 8:00 a.m. for routine work. During pleasurable, exciting living, "time flies"; during periods of boredom, "time drags."

Obsessive-compulsive patients tend to be scrupulously aware of the exact time and its passage. Highly anxious or depressed patients tend to feel that time is passing slowly and consequently underestimate the hour. A manic patient may want his lunch an hour after breakfast, whereas a severely depressed one may have trouble believing it is time to eat when a nurse brings his lunch. Most schizophrenic patients reveal a profound temporal disorientation as to time when agitated or severely withdrawn, but even those in catatonic stupor retain a degree of deeper awareness. Other schizophrenic patients have a highly personalized, subtle sense of the meaning of time, difficult for the interviewer to grasp.

A disturbance of the concept of the passage of time is one of the earliest indicators of organic brain disease, or impending delirious states, in patients who are suffering from toxic, metabolic, or other types of encephalopathy.

Place: Disturbance of orientation as to place is indicative of a serious organic brain disease or schizophrenia. The delirious patient may mistake the hospital for a prison or a torture chamber, and in his efforts to escape may injure himself unless adequate treatment is instituted promptly. Patients with advanced chronic brain disease may cheerfully think that they are at home, instead of in the hospital or other institution. Schizophrenic patients who disregard external reality to an advanced degree may say that the hospital is either a cherished abode of some type or a chamber of horrors, depending on the nature of their delusional system.

Person: Disorientation in the sphere of personal identity is seen following cerebral trauma or seizures and in amnesic, fugue-like states. Although some schizophrenic patients insist that they are heroic or notorious celebrities, godlike creatures or demons, most of them still maintain an awareness of their personal identity. Loss of this knowledge is seen only occasionally in patients with chronic organic brain disease and then only in very advanced states.

Although the *I* of self-identity is regarded as the only certain anchor in the subject's universe, wide variations in awareness of the self occur within the limits of normal self-perception, as well as in neurotic and psychotic conditions.

When severe disappointments and unbearable sufferings make withdrawal and isolation seem necessary, feelings of depersonalization arise in which even normal subjects for a time deny the reality of their experiences. When the privations, humiliations and tortures suffered by inmates of a Nazi concentration camp reached a limit of tolerance, the victims began to feel as though they were remote witnesses of another person's nightmare, and existed in a state in which their own identity was only dimly retained. A strongly integrated and resilient individual can again accept "external" reality once the extreme stresses have passed, whereas with the development of neurotic or psychotic processes, amnesias and feelings of greater or lesser depersonalization may become progressive and persistent. This progression may appear abrupt in the case of a person who suddenly "snaps" and who assumes a secretly desired identity while in a dissociated state. But when, for example, the full history of the puritanical minister who disappeared from a small, conservative village and was later found to be living as a relatively unrestrained Bohemian under a different name in a nearby city was obtained, it became apparent that the individual had been living under many stresses for months or years before he more or less deliberately decided on a complete change of life style. In schizophrenia the withdrawal and self-isolation are particularly marked and often colored by bizarre and fragmented symbolisms, compensatory grandiosities and by distortions in the patient's image of the shape, movement, weight and consistency of the various parts of his own body.

Interpersonal Relationships

There exists in everyone a tendency to invest others with "projected" and generalized identities derived from previous experiences and evaluations. As a superficial instance, all clerics are treated with the uneasy awe or resentment one may accord his own minister, or all aged folk are treated a little like one's ancestors. A patient will therefore feel toward his physician a mixture of the enforced reliance and covert anxiety with which he formerly regarded his parents or their surrogates, but marked exaggerations and deviations of attitude may also be observed in the clinical examination. Thus, the neurotic or depressed adult may become excessively dependent and demand as much of the physician as a helpless infant does of its mother—or, conversely, the patient may be as fearful and hostile as a rejected child. So also patients in schizoid and paranoid states may regard the examiner as an enemy or attribute to him an infinite variety of other fantasied roles.

Affective State

The patient's mood and emotional state at the time of examination can, with practice, be fairly accurately surmised from both his verbal and nonverbal behavior. The easy, almost *laissez-faire* indifference (attitude approaching equanimity) of the conversion neurotic stands in marked contrast to the strained voice, troubled expression and restless tension of the patient with free-floating anxiety or impending panic. The stooped posture, drawn facies and slow monotone of the depressed patient are expressive of his self-deprecatory, melancholic ideation and are distinguishable from the dream-like, aloof self-preoccupation of the schizoid who surrounds himself with barriers to empathy and effective communication with the examiner. True euphoria in psychiatric disorders is relatively rare despite frequent references to it in case descriptions. In many instances what is called "manic" euphoria is not really a state of uninhibited elation, but rather an uneasy flight from one rapidly discarded fantasy and activity to another. So also, admixtures of attitudes, affects and transference relationships such as suspiciousness, irritability, truculence and other variously toned reactions may be noted in the context of the interview.

The patient's affective responses (feeling tones accompanying an idea) should be noted, and sometimes tested, during the interview, for appropriateness in type and degree and for range of expression. A disturbance of affect is seen in most patients with various neurotic conditions, for example, the classical "la belle indifference" of the patient with conversion symptoms, the dramatic affective responses displayed by the hysteric, or the controlled affectivity of the obsessive-compulsive. Even less appropriate responses may occur—for example, the patient's smiling while he discusses a tragic event or appearing sad while he discusses an ostensibly happy one. These emotional responses can be relevant in type but inappropriate in degree, as evidenced by the manic patient's becoming hilarious over only a slightly humorous matter.

Disorders of affect and mood are also manifest in various depressive states, and manic-depressive psychoses. Schizophrenic patients' affectivity may range between blunted, shallow affects to bizarre and extreme emotional displays during the examination.

Special Symptoms

These include compulsions, obsessions, phobias, fugues, transient disturbances of consciousness or other significant phenomena. Topical beliefs which in our society cannot be labelled "delusions" may range from "normal" economic or social dogmatism to superstitions or mystic preoccupations not uncommonly encountered in the general populace. Illusional experiences may range from occasional misidentifications of objects and events in anxiety states to the frequent misinterpretations of environmental stimuli. However, when beliefs become bizarre, pervasive, fixed, widely deviant from accepted norms in the patient's own cultural group, and destructive in their consequences, they may properly be termed delusional and, if organized into a persecutory system, paranoiac.

Insight

This is best recorded as a statement of the patient's spontaneous formulations as to the nature, etiology and proper treatment of his illness. All forms and combinations of such statements will be encountered. One patient may insist that his symptoms are due entirely to organic disease; another may profess the same belief yet admit the influence of "emotional factors" in his illness. Or, a third may volunteer that "I know it's just my nerves, doctor," yet mean by "nervousness" an actual physical disorder of the nervous system treatable only by drugs, diets or surgery. Even more deceptively, a patient may come to the physician with made-to-order psychologic "explanations" of his self-styled "neurosis" (usually in the form of superficial cliches derived from books on inspirational or "popular" psychology), and then proceed to use these empty formulas to befog any real progress toward self-understanding. An intelligent "sociopath" may be capable of pertinent and penetrating self-evaluations, yet rest content with such empty verbalization of "insight" and stolidly refuse to utilize this knowledge in planning, let alone executing, any constructive reorientations and redirections of his behavior. The person who makes satisfactory improvements under therapy without necessarily verbalizing his reasons for doing so exhibits more self-realization than the devotee of psychiatry whose vast "self-knowledge" remains solely within the realm of verbalization. A patient's "insight," therefore, should be described in behavioral rather than merely semantic terms, and evaluated objectively rather than according to theoretical preconceptions.

THE PHYSICAL EXAMINATION

Adequate physical, neurologic and laboratory examinations are indispensable parts of a complete psychiatric study and must be supplemented when necessary by roentgenologic, electroencephalographic and other special diagnostic procedures. This seems obvious, yet many a patient hospitalized after a traumatic experience for "hysterical coma" has been found to have a cerebral hemorrhage, and many a carelessly diagnosed "organ neurosis" has been proved, on medical or surgical examination, to have a pathologic substrate in actual tissue disease. But the diagnostic error in the reverse direction may also be cited: character neuroses treated interminably and futilely by vitamins, diets and "changes of climate"; thyroidectomies for anxiety or panic states; or appendices, gallbladders and other more or less expendable abdominal organs relinquished uselessly by masochistic patients who seek the surgeon's magic as a cure for purely hypochondriac discomforts and dysfunctions. The psychiatric interviewer, then, must be as competent and careful in diagnosing organic disease in his patients as the internist and surgeon should be in detecting neurotic disturbances in theirs; indeed, all physicians must be capable of dealing with the entire body and its total behavior.

Psychiatrically Significant Aspects of the Physical Examination

During the physical examination, observations of psychiatric significance may easily be made: e.g., excessive shyness, exhibitionism or erotic hypersensitivity, tattoo-marks, poor oral and ungual hygiene, tobacco stains, drug rashes, evidences of excessive scratching or more specific self injury, and the marks of frequent hypodermic or intravenous injections.

THE NEUROLOGIC EXAMINATION

The neurologic examination may confirm the functional nature of various professed disabilities. For example, it may disclose: (1) that the extent and distribution of a paralysis or a localized anesthesia cannot be attributed solely to an organic lesion, (2) that vision is present even when without the patient's knowledge his "only good eye" is blinded by a lens, (3) that speech becomes confused when the patient's words are electronically relayed with a quarter-second delay to a professedly "deaf" ear, or (4) that a supposedly monoplegic arm "falls" through an arc so arranged that the recumbent patient at one stage unwittingly lifts it against gravity. In general, too, the patient's conduct may reveal resentment, suspiciousness, deliberate attempts at malingering, or other affects and attitudes that confirm previous inferences derived from the history and mental status examination. Finally, various tests of perception, grasp, integration, understanding and communication are of both neurologic and psychiatric significance, and may be briefly outlined as follows.

Tests of Apperceptive-Expressive Functions (Psychomotor Aphasia)

We may first consider a relatively simple example requiring interpersonal communication. If a patient, during the course of physical examination, is asked by the physician "Is the pressure of my fingers on your abdomen painful?" his reply will obviously be contingent on a number of factors. First, he must be interested in the question, else there will be no incentive to attend to it. Second, he must hear the words or read them from the physician's lips, else there is no meaningful stimulus requiring a specific response. Third, he must recognize the "content" of the question in terms of past experience, integrate its meaning with the relevance of whatever sensations are coming from his abdomen, and then evaluate the significance of the entire situation. Even then, his reply is still dependent on his ability to speak or write words with generally accepted meanings, or at least to express by grimace or gesture his interest in, his understanding of, and his response to the physician's investigation.

Similarly, the functions of interpersonal communications may be analyzed into (a) the volitional, (b) the apperceptive (including sensory, comparative, integrative and interpretative processes), and (c) the expressive (including speech, writing and nonverbal communication). Volition is fundamental to all behavior; but, especially in patients with possible central nervous system disease, an examination of other determinants of communicative function often yields results which have direct clinical significance. Wherever indicated, these determinants may be partially isolated and tested according to the following schema.

Apperceptive Processes in Relation to Spoken Response

Aural Perception. Depending on circumstances varying from the presence of coma to that of communication only in highly specialized fields, the patient can be asked questions ranging in complexity from "Do you hear me?" or "What is your name?" to "What do you think of the new space program?" Allowing for factors such as the patient's interest, intelligence and disturbances in the expressive arc of the response, his replies may indicate sensory deafness, deficiencies of verbal understanding ("aphasia in inner language") or total abolition of auditory apperception despite intact hearing (auditory agnosia). Similar tests of auditory perception may require the patient to identify nonverbal stimuli such as a buzzer, a whistle, a cough, or the pitch, timbre, rhythm and melodic themes of familiar musical selections (amusia).

Visual Perception. The patient is asked to reply vocally to written questions or to interpret printed paragraphs. These tests can be refined by presenting the material in inverted form or mixed sequence and noting the efficiency with which the patient rearranges it, or in what ways he reveals disturbances in understanding written language such as alexia. Similar tests may be made with pictures or incomplete drawings which uncover asymbolia, or with the verbal identification of familiar objects such as pencil or a watch which disclose visual agnosia.

Stereognosia. This is tested by asking the patient to name objects such as coins or Braille letters solely by touch.

Olfactory Perception. To test the integrity of olfaction, ask the patient to identify common odors (avoid irritating ones such as ammonia which also stimulate the fifth nerve.)

Gustatory Perception. Ask the patient to recognize common tastes, such as salt, chocolate or vinegar.

In the above tests the organization of perceptions in the three most important sensory modalities (hearing, sight, and feel) and the two lesser ones (smell and taste) have been apposed to spoken responses elicited from the patient, but all of these responses may be distorted or abolished by disturbances in speech expression (motor aphasia). Such disturbances may consist of blockings and obliterations, uncontrolled verbalization (logorrhea), deviated expression (paraphasia), mixed or reversed words (jargonaphasia, streptosymbolia), perseveration of words or phrases (verbigeration), or the unaccustomed and not consciously intended insertion of obscene or profane interjections or inept jokes (*Witzelsucht*). Inverted sentence structure, grammatical errors, and other deviations of verbal expression are likewise significant. Sometimes the organic cerebral lesions revealed, and in part localized, by the disturbances in communicative functions here outlined affect only a language acquired by the patient in later life and leave relatively intact one learned in childhood. Furthermore, some of these aberrations may improve or disappear when the patient is asked to sing the words of a song; in this case the verbal expressions are bolstered by deep-seated rhythmic and melodic associations.

Apperceptive Processes in Relation to Written Responses

The procedures outlined above may be repeated in each of the sensory modalities, with instructions that the patient now write out his responses. If this is impossible because of a paralysis of the dominant arm, the other may be used, or the patient may spell out his answer by selecting words or letters from a print-box.

Apperceptive Processes in Relation to Nonverbal Responses

To test these various sensory apperceptions request the patient to hum or whistle a melody, to mimic fear, to perform certain successive movements, to draw diagrams or images, to point to selected objects and then use them properly. Disturbances in such motor manipulations are grouped under the term *apraxia* and may have prefrontal, parietal and cerebellar components.

Apperceptive Processes in Relation to Nonevaluative Activity

Finally, in severe organic cerebral deficiencies semi-automatic processes involving lesser degrees of spontaneous integration and organization may be tested. Thus, the patient may be directed, in any way available, to repeat words or read aloud from print or Braille, to take dictation or copy writing, or simply to mimic the motions of the examiner.

Evaluation of Tests

It is evident that the tests here described are multiple, time-consuming and unavoidably lacking in precision. Although general disturbances in communication may be correlated with the functions of special regions of the brain (e.g., visual perception in the occipital lobe, auditory perception in the temporal gyri, space perception in the parietal region, motor speech and "dynamic visual field" in the prefrontal cortex), such correlations cannot be anatomically exact because all parts of the brain are utilized in the highly complex and interdependent processes of speech. Conversely, any brain lesion may produce disturbances, however subtle, in all the modalities of inner perception and outer expression. Even though the tests outlined are not often useful for exact neurological localization, they may serve to reveal *functional* deficiencies in communication that might otherwise be overlooked and which need to be considered in the psychiatric diagnosis and prognosis of patients with central nervous system disease. When such deficiencies are revealed, they may be more closely delimited by more specialized procedures.

DRUGS AS AIDS IN THE PSYCHIATRIC INTERVIEW

Sometimes a patient's anxieties, inhibitions and repressions are so great that despite the psychiatrist's every effort the initial exploratory maneuvers reveal insufficient information or increase the patient's tensions. Such reactions are relatively frequent in acute traumatic neuroses (e.g., after catastrophic accidents, floods, fires, earthquakes) in which the victim, numbed and overwhelmed by an accumulation of stresses, could not bring himself to reexplore his experiences, accept the physician's psychotherapeutic aid, and thus obtain surcease from doubts, fears, and terrors. In such cases and in some depressions or borderline schizophrenias, the use of drugs that temporarily remove inhibitions may give the patient a transient, welcome relief from persistent agitation and also an opportunity for affective catharsis and transference expression. Various drugs may be used for these purposes: alcohol by mouth, Pentothal sodium or Sodium Amytal by intravenous injection, or Valium intravenously. Usually, Sodium Amytal is preferable for general use because of its relative safety, ease of administration, and effectiveness.

Contraindications to Amytal Hypnosis

These may be grouped as follows:

Physical. Sodium Amytal should not be given intravenously if the patient has acute infections; serious cardiovascular, pulmonary, renal, hepatic or skin diseases; blood dyscrasias; marked malnutrition; or (since it is a strongly alkaline solution) impending alkalosis. The usual dose of 500 mgm. in 10% sterile water should be reduced in the aged or in those with organic central nervous system disease to avoid excessive effects. Affective furors, catatonic excitements, and other agitated states in which the sedative action of the drug may be helpful should be carefully differentiated by clinical and chemical studies from chloral, bromide, barbiturate, or other drug delirium, in which an added dose of Amytal intravenously might have serious consequences. Finally, a few individuals with an unpredictable idiosyncrasy may develop, cardiovascular and respiratory depression manifested by cyanosis, dyspnea, irregularity of the pulse, and syncope after the intravenous injection of small quantities. If these signs impend, or the patient's diastolic pressure drops more than 15 mm. of mercury, the administration of the drug should be stopped immediately; if recovery does not then occur promptly or shock threatens, intravenous fluids containing one ampule of Levophed (4 ml.) should be started and the patient's airway kept open. Such adverse reactions are rare, but must be met promptly.

Psychologic. Except in the acute stages of catastrophic or "traumatic" neuroses, little is generally accomplished by drug narcosis that could not also be achieved by anamnestic and therapeutic interviews conducted without its use. As noted, Amytal or other drugs may aid in history-taking and in the modification or removal of symptoms, but in most cases employing pharmacologic adjuvants for these purposes is contraindicated. Patients who have not been adequately orientated by preliminary therapy or whose neurotic defenses are too rapidly threatened by these techniques may disclaim the memory or the significance of their behavior under Amytal, even though the "Amytal interview" produced relevant data or temporarily reduced their symptoms. Indeed, some patients distort the whole procedure by claiming that it demonstrated the organic nature of their illness since symptomatic relief could occur only if drugs were administered. In the preparation of such patients for drug narcosis special care must be taken to prevent these rationalizations, but despite every explanation before and after the treatment, the patient may maintain this view and insist that therapy involve further drug administration. In fact, patients who have experienced relief from neurotic tensions under alcohol, barbiturates, or other drugs may seek out the drugs for themselves and eventually become addicted. Also, patients whose deep longings for passivity and protective domination are more or less consciously satisfied by drug narcosis may form an attachment to the procedure (or directly to the physician) and remain fixed in an altered but hardly preferable neurotic pattern. Conversely, patients with latent paranoid tendencies may become suspicious, hostile and recriminative—a possibility that necessitates the presence of a witness to refute the patient's retrospective falsifications about what occurred during the interview. Finally, anamnestic insights and therapeutic gains achieved during narcosis are evanescent unless they are reviewed, accepted, and applied by the patient in actual life situations; but when the prognosis for making behavioral changes is promising, the narcosis technique offers no lasting advantage.

Clinical Applications of Narcosis

Despite these important reservations Amytal or other types of narcosis, when used judiciously with selected patients, may be of aid in psychiatric diagnosis and prognosis:

CASE 17:   Use of Sodium Amytal as an ancillary anamnestic technique. A 21-year-old unmarried Jewish girl was admitted to the hospital with a history, furnished by companions, that during the previous three weeks she had become uncommunicative and resistant to care and had occasionally complained of being "followed" and "slowly poisoned." Since the patient had apparently developed her illness while en route from Europe to Chicago, where her distant relatives knew little about her, and since she refused to answer questions in any foreign language spoken by various members of the staff, Sodium Amytal was used in an attempt to obtain a working history. The first few drops of the injection produced a remarkable effect: the patient, previously suspicious and resistive, dropped her reserve and began to sigh and then to cry softly. Soon she became relatively alert and responsive, and thereafter, in a polite manner and with normal inflection and affectivity, answered in good English any question put to her. This period of responsiveness lasted for half an hour, after which she tired, withdrew her interest, and gradually resumed her previous evasiveness and mute stolidity. The administration of additional Sodium Anytal at this point had little or no effect other than to induce drowsiness or sleep. But when an injection was given the next day, another period of rapport and productivity was induced. In this way it was possible to obtain a detailed and highly significant account of emotional conflicts that had precipitated her present illness. These consisted of early familial separations, and, finally, her seduction and desertion by a man en route.

CASE 18:   Use of Amytal to confirm significant data. A 40-year-old engineer while away from his wife for several months on a professional assignment had an extramarital affair and returned home contrite and guilt-ridden. Soon afterward, he was informed by a jealous neighbor that his wife had been seen in the company of other men in suspicious circumstances. When he challenged her to give a complete accounting of herself, she denied any current unfaithfulness; however, in covert retaliation she also insisted on telling him "the whole truth once and for all," and described two casual sexual liaisons that had occurred long before she had met her husband. This drove him into a state of agitation which threatened his business and social status as well as his marriage.

After a few interviews the patient began to see that what he dreaded was not his wife's unfaithfulness, but the breakdown of a system of fantasied personal superiority which had begun with his parents' indulgence, his own unusual success at school, and later his dominance of his familial and social group. As these fantasies were put in a more realistic setting, his severe depression lessened and the crisis was averted. However, one crucial issue remained: since his wife had claimed that she was a virgin at the time of their marriage and had obviously lied to him, could she be lying now, and could he have further trust in her or in anyone else?

It is possible that months of psychotherapy would have resolved this rationalization and much else that it represented. Meanwhile, however, his professional career would have suffered and his wife and children would have been in a prolonged state of disruptive insecurity. The therapist interviewed the wife and was convinced that she had been truthful, but he also knew that the husband would continue to doubt her. An alternative plan was therefore proposed, to which all agreed. The wife would be given Sodium Amytal (regarded by the patient as a "truth serum") and the patient would be permitted to question her directly in any way he desired—*provided that he agreed not to continue to doubt the veracity of whatever she said.*

The technique was successful. Under Amytal, the wife repeated convincingly what she had told her husband previously, and because the patient now wanted desperately to believe her, he did. Only two more interviews were necessary; twelve years later he and his wife were still attributing—somewhat inaccurately—his complete recovery and their reunion to the trial of the Amytal administration.

CASE 19: Amytal as an aid in differential diagnosis. A 41-year-old married woman was brought to the hospital because, according to the family, during the previous three years she had become progressively more forgetful, slovenly, confused, irritable and, more recently, almost uncontrollably quarrelsome and aggressive. Neurologic examination revealed bilateral rapid nystagmoid movements, pallor of the temporal portions of both optic discs and positive Hoffman reflexes. The mental status, moreover, showed signs indicative of organic cortical aphasia: the patient had difficulty expressing herself and contorted her features while casting about for what she wanted to say. She was confused about the time and sequence of past events. She answered "Yes" or "Fine" to evade misunderstood, though simple, questions, and followed her statements with a doubtful "Is that right?" or a misplaced "Hold the phone!" She frequently stated, "There is something in my head that does not allow things to come through clearly." Her memory was deficient in all spheres, as were her replies to simple tests of calculation, association, orientation and general information. Whenever an attempt was made to obtain some account of her illness she replied with "You can worm these things out of me. Go on asking questions."

A week after admission, she was given 0.3 gm. of Sodium Amytal intravenously. At first she became combative, talked rapidly, and even tried to pull the stethoscope from the intern. However, she also grew talkative and during the next half hour gave an account of her history. This was clear and detailed, and dealt frankly with early family and school experiences, occupational adjustments, various love affairs previous to her marriage, and sexual and economic dissatisfactions thereafter. Next she discussed what she thought was the precipitating cause of her illness—"overwork and aggravation." Physical exhaustion had resulted from having to devote the last three years of her life to taking care of her blind and aged mother while trying to run the family business. Under the effects of Amytal she spoke rapidly and surely, without the pseudoaphasic difficulties that had characterized her previous interviews. When the effects of the drug had worn off, however, the patient resumed her previous mannerisms, taciturnity and uncooperativeness.

It was evident that she suffered from an Alzheimer syndrome, but that disabilities arising from depression and withdrawal were added to her organic defects. This was confirmed by the favorable influence of two more Amytal interviews and follow-up psychotherapy.

REFERENCES

1. Freedman, A. M. and Kaplan, H. I. (Eds.): *Diagnosing Mental Illness*. New York, Science House, 1973.
2. Masserman, J. H.: *The Optimal Psychiatric Interview*. Fort Lee, N.J., Behavior Science Tape Library, 1973.
3. Sands, W. L.: Psychiatric history and mental status. *In* Freedman, A. M. and Kaplan, H. I. (Eds.): *Comprehensive Textbook of Psychiatry*. Baltimore, Williams & Wilkins, 1967 (pp. 499–508).

Chapter 5

SPECIAL ASPECTS OF THE PSYCHIATRIC EXAMINATION

THE PSYCHIATRIC HISTORY AS MENTAL STATUS

It is sometimes difficult for those trained to regard historical accounts as immutable data to appreciate more subtle aspects of the psychiatric interview. In the sense of its Greek root, "history" itself is not merely a chronologic account of physical or human events, but a logical evaluation and appraisal of such data in terms of their meaning and significance. So also, the psychiatric "history," as obtained from a patient, is primarily significant as a *communicative interplay between examiner and patient.* Operationally, *all* the material obtained in such interviews is necessarily "true" in that it reflects the patient's current behavior patterns or "mental status." This can be clarified by the following examples:

A patient with chronic alcoholic encephalopathy (Korsakoff psychosis) is confined in a state institution, yet every day he invents different stories about travels, sexual adventures, or other fanciful experiences in which he claims to be participating. Under such circumstances, the information furnished by the patient will, of course, be correctly interpreted not as "fact" but as symbolic wishfulness distorted in time, place and content by (a) organic cerebral dysfunctions and (b) his attempts to overcompensate through superficial cheerfulness and grandiosity for an insistent and disquieting sense of his own growing inadequacies.

A phobic child may give a highly colored account of the many-toothed, roaring, horrendous creatures that lurk about his bed at night. From such descriptions the child psychiatrist can conclude that the child has many fears including markedly phobic misconceptions of dogs or cats; i.e., he accepts the child's exaggerated fears as "facts," without necessarily tracing down the remote possibility that the child's parents really keep saber-toothed tigers roaming about the house.

Conversely, a "normal" anamnesis can be viewed as misleading:

For instance, a patient may dwell at length upon the devotion shown him by his parents, the beauties of his childhood environment, and the delights of his early experiences. Such memories may or may not be accurate, but what is "true" in many cases is that the patient is exhibiting a flight from current boredom or conflicts into regressive longings for times retrospectively judged happier, while simultaneously making a bid for the examiner's regard for him as a loyal and faithful son.

Or, the patient may give a consistent history to the effect that his parents and siblings were tyrannical, that he was mishandled at school, exploited by his employers, and misunderstood and mistreated by previous physicians. Again, such statements are usually both reflections of and defenses against his current feelings of rejection, suspicion, and reactive aggression toward all persons of authority, including the examiner.

Properly to interpret interview material then, it must be remembered that a subject will furnish only such data as he (a) dynamically selects to remember or invent, (b) is prepared to face, and (c) wants his examiner to hear. Yet for these very reasons every anamnesis gives "objective" and significant information about the patient, whether or not the "biographic" material is "true" in any other sense.

THE PSYCHIATRIC HISTORY AS INITIAL THERAPY

By laying the ground work for rapport or "transference" relationships the anamnestic interview presents the examiner with the first opportunity to initiate therapy. As noted, the patient should find the interviewer to be a kindly, interested, trustworthy, and tolerant person, who gives an early impression of being informed, experienced, and capable of helping, whether the patient conceives his problems to be medical, personal, or environmental. An inhibited, ineffectual "passivity" on the examiner's part, an obsessive routine of history-taking with disregard of the patient's sensibilities, a covertly condemnatory attitude, premature reassurances or stereotyped "formulations" calculated to impress the patient, or other failures in technique indicate lack of experience and refinement in interviewing. Moreover, they prejudice development of the history and the pursuit of effective therapy. An extreme but instructive example is the following:

CASE 20:   The dynamics of a psychophysiologic reaction (ocular ptosis). A large, raw-boned 46-year-old Catholic woman came to the hospital with a persistent ptosis of both eye lids of some six months' duration. Ophthalmic, physical, and neurologic examinations showed only normal findings, and since it was observed that the ptosis varied markedly with her emotional state, she was sent to the Psychiatric Clinic. Here a "psychoanalytically oriented" resident, himself under analysis, interviewed the patient and obtained the following story:

The patient stated that she had supported her husband in idleness and had taken all responsibility for raising their two children for the last twenty years. She had become quite resigned to her "sacrifices for their sake." Six months previous to the interview, however, her husband, after two days of unexplained absence, had been brought home seriously ill with pneumonia, and the patient had "nursed him day and night for a week until I could hardly keep my eyes open." A few days later, an actual ptosis of her eyelids developed and had persisted until she came to the hospital. The patient also confided that she had never experienced orgasm until after her husband's recent illness, when his potency had seemed to increase. However, she "disliked" the "nervous feeling" of orgasm, and considered its occurrence as another sign of the same "nervous disease" that was causing the paralysis of her eyelids. In her past history she laid considerable stress on the fact that her revered mother had died when the patient was 7, and that thereafter her life had been made miserable by her father and an unsympathetic older brother.

With this bare "case material" in hand, the inexperienced therapist proceeded to "formulate the case" as follows: Because of reactive hostility to her father, the patient had formed an inverted Oedipus complex in early life; i.e., she wished to castrate him and become masculine herself so that she could preempt her father's place in her mother's affections. This had formed the basis for a latent homosexuality that had caused the patient to grow up with a masculine habitus, to marry a weak, ineffectual, effeminate husband, to "repress" feminine orgasm, and to assume the male role in their marital and occupational relationships. However, when the patient's ambivalently hostile wishes toward her husband—a father-surrogate—seemed about to be fulfilled by his death, the patient, in self-punitive expiation of her guilt, symbolically castrated herself by a displaced dysfunction of her eyes as testicle-equivalents. Thus, again turned feminine, she could permit herself to enjoy intercourse and proceeded to do so, though with enough residual guilt to make it necessary for her to deny complete fulfillment.

It need hardly be pointed out that with limited anamnestic material, these "psychodynamic formulations" could be nothing but pure *a priori* speculations. Furthermore, even if they were justified at the deepest level of analysis, they were irrelevant for immediate diagnostic purposes and might lead to gross psychotherapeutic errors. The latter danger was made evident by later interviews with the patient which revealed the following:

The patient was a querulous, emotionally labile woman of limited intelligence who had, quite early in life, acquired the pattern of seeking sympathy and help from others by trying to impress them with her own self-sacrificing and deserving nature. She had given this version to the ophthalmologist and, later, had furnished an even more appealing story to the psychiatric resident. Actually, other informants made clear that she had been overindulged by her mother during early childhood, and had interpreted her father's attempts at normal corrective discipline as cruelty. To escape this she had married an easy-going and tolerant individual whom she tyrannized by nagging accusations and threats of sexual frustration. After a decade, he finally rebelled and threatened divorce, from which she dissuaded him by emphasizing their Catholicism. Then, to hurt his pride, she began working half-time and saved what little

money she made "for her own future." She was deeply dependent on her husband, and was jealous of her daughters, to whom he was devoted. When the
oldest daughter became illegitimately pregnant, the patient's husband forgave
the daughter and promised to keep the child; however, during his illness the
patient arranged to have the daughter illegally aborted and then told her husband how she herself had viewed the operation and seen the bloody fetus
extruded. In a rage the husband denounced the patient and, among other
curses, invoked the saints to strike her blind in punishment for her lack of maternal feeling. He then left home for two days, returning only because he needed
rest for an acute upper respiratory infection. Another quarrel ensued, which
ended with the patient in a hysterical stupor, from which she emerged with "par-
alyzed" eyelids. Conscience-stricken because his "curse had come true," the
husband forgave the patient and redoubled his attentions to her in her thoroughly dramatized martyrdom. To encourage this more gratifying attitude on
his part, the patient had permitted him a sexual freedom more satisfactory to
both of them—ergo the "sexual history" given the first interviewer.

In the light of this reformulation, treatment proceeded along fairly
evident lines. Both the patient and the husband were informed of the functional nature of the illness. Their current recriminatons, guilts and hostilities were ventilated and readjusted by relatively direct discussions. Next,
the patient's ward routine, hospital contacts, and activities were arranged
so that she began to yearn to participate in them with eyes wide open
rather than isolate herself in a half-blind retreat. "Reading" exercises or
other devices that might concentrate her attention on her blindness were
avoided; rather, she was assured that with self-understanding and control
her vision would rapidly improve. Finally, with the help of the family,
marital relationships were reoriented so that the patient was likely to obtain
greater attention and security through more mature wifely and maternal
behavior than through covert aggressivity, regression and neurotic illness.
At no time were any symbolic "interpretations" or analytic formulations
given her about the illness. Instead, her symptoms were quite frankly
referred to as "unfortunate habits" acquired when her judgment and responses were suboptimal, but could be improved for her own benefit. This
seemingly "superficial" therapy, as applied by the entire ward personnel
with skill and depth of understanding, produced tangible results. Within
two weeks the ptosis disappeared and in another week the patient returned
home. Two years later she and her family reported that she had remained
"cured" and that their relationships had never been better.

Commentary

Heuristically, no man can ever know the "real" universe, since he can
sense, classify and "interpret" the *data* which are given him only within the

limits of his own capacities and interests. In the sciences of human behavior, the perception and interpretation of another's inner experiences as compared with one's own variable reactions is especially complex. Sweeping theories which purport to explain the matrical multidimensionality of human behavior, however oracularly asserted, are too often regarded as eternally established. Clinicians should therefore not perpetuate current misconceptions, prejudices, and errors by reading them into the case history and formulation; instead, these should be as factual and therapeutically relevant as skill and conscience can make them. Then and then only can we erect a relatively sound foundation upon which to build, alter, and improve our clinical superstructure of rationale and practice.

Progressive Distortions

These, too, must be guarded against. As an example, the "case history" for some "clinical seminars" may be a bewildering compound of: (1) what the patient can or wishes to remember about his own behavior; (2) what he elects to tell the interviewer taking the "history"; (3) what the latter hears or understands; (4) what he then selects to record in his notes ; (5) what he subsequently adds or deletes in order to "integrate his findings"; (6) what the interviewer's supervisor changes, eliminates or reformulates before the "material" is presented at the seminar; (7) what each conferee hears, as filtered through his own sensitivities, preferences and prejudices; and finally (8) how the conferees severally "formulate the case," according to their individual biases and interests. Too often, any resemblence to the original is obscured in this melee of successive drawings, quarterings and extractions.

Individual Variations

Biographic distortions are not solely artefacts of the mechanics of group presentation and discussion; the errors of individual prejudice, though more subtle, may be just as pervasive.

An instance of how preconceptions affect observations of "reality" is afforded by the study of R. S. Kaufman who tested theories of "psychokinesis" (the influence of "mental set" on external events) by having four believers in this phenomenon and four nonbelievers throw dice while attempting to influence the results by mental concentration. A camera and calculator which recorded the throws showed that the dice had come up in exact accord with the mathematical probabilities; however, the believers observed "data" that "proved" the theories, whereas the score sheets of the scoffers, with equal significance, showed readings directly contrary to those wished for. Another instance of the influence of personal bias is illustrated by an analyst's assertion in an open meeting that "patients never dream in color"; inquiry revealed that the analyst was color-blind.

Another example is an experiment performed on himself by Dr. L.K., a highly respected psychoanalyst: He had observed that his trainees' reports of their patients' psychodynamic patterns of unconscious motivation and defense were often unmistakably similar to those of the trainee's own personality. Dr. K. justifiably wondered whether even he as well as his "best analyzed" students might not still be projecting their own difficulties onto their patients, accounting for the strangely syncretic results of their own clinical viewpoints. Dr. K. proceeded to test his hypothesis. With their consent, he made sound recordings of his patients' analytic sessions, and, as usual, he took notes. Without consulting the recordings, he pretended that he was again a student and from these notes prepared written summaries and formulations of two weeks of analytic work as though he were actually going to present it to a former "control analyst" for comment.

Then, he put these reports and formulations aside for several weeks. Finally, taking the role of the control analyst, he compared his prepared formulations with a review of the patient's tape-recorded verbalizations. He learned to his chagrin that, notwithstanding his efforts at objectivity and despite his long training and experience, he had fallen into some of the same errors he had suspected in his students. In effect, he had permitted his own biases and preferences to creep into both his selection and formulation of the clinical material. In one instance, he had even cast his presentation so as to render it more acceptable to the well-liked former "control analyst."

If one of the most capable observers in this field can fall into such inductive and evaluative errors, those less experienced must be circumspect indeed.

REFERENCES

1. Berger, M. M. (Ed.): *Videotape Techniques in Psychiatric Training and Treatment,* New York, Brunner/Mazel, 1970.
2. Masserman, J. H.: *Videotaped Illustrations of Special Techniques in Examining Psychiatric Patients.* Distributed by Veterans Administration Hospital, Downey, Illinois.
3. Scheflen A. E. and Scheflen, Alice: *Body Language and Social Order.* Englewood Cliffs, N.J., Prentice-Hall, 1972.

Chapter 6

INTRODUCTION TO PSYCHOLOGICAL TESTING

This chapter will offer a general orientation and brief background material for psychodiagnostic testing, highlighting its rationale and utility for the psychiatric interviewer.

Psychiatry and psychology have a common scientific heritage. For example, one of the greatest 19th century psychiatrists, Kraepelin, worked with Wundt, the father of experimental psychology. Williams James, whose work on consciousness in the 1890s is an intellectual masterpiece still not outdated, and whose theories provided a basis for the social psychology of Mead and Cooley, was a physician and a philosopher as well as a psychologist. Sigmund Freud often referred to the theoretical aspects of psychoanalysis as metapsychology. The experimental neurophysiological work of Kurt Goldstein, Paul Schilder, and Lauretta Bender provided a necessary background for neuropsychological testing. As Sargent and Mayman emphasize, Hermann Rorschach was a Swiss psychiatrist; Henry Murray, who developed the Thematic Apperception Test, had a medical degree, and the word-association method was elaborated by Jung. The work of Rollo May on anxiety and existentialism, that of Cattell on testing, and the contributions of many other psychologists have enriched the theory and practice of psychiatry.

Any single testing procedure can seldom furnish a complete answer to a diagnostic or therapeutic problem. Even in physical medicine the physician must differentiate between the clinical condition and the biochemical or other abnormality which may or may not produce symptoms and disease. Psychological tests are useful adjuncts to the case history, mental status examination, laboratory studies, and all other factual knowledge necessary for understanding a patient and for the application of sound clinical judgment.

PRINCIPLES OF TESTING

A psychological test is usually defined as a directed sample of varied stimuli selected and organized on an experimental or experiential basis to elicit information about mental functions and personality traits. The results are scored according to established criteria and interpreted according to empiric norms and the psychologist's clinical judgment.

Validity

Validity refers to the capability of the test to measure what it purports to evaluate. Fundamentally, validation depends upon obtaining agreement between at least two empirical types of data which are derived from at least two different sources—for example, the comparison of a score on a test to another independent criterion of performance. Specifically, the four types of validation are:

(1) *Predictive Validity*, or the capability and power of the test to predict a designated outcome. For example, intelligence or aptitude tests should be helpful in predicting a student's scholastic performance, and neuropsychological tests are of value in predicting the degree of the patient's recovery following a stroke.

(2) *Concurrent Validity*, or the capability of the test to estimate present performance. Concurrent validity for a test should be measured when it is offered as an alternative for another test or as a substitute for information derived from other sources. Usually, concurrent validity is dependent upon high correlations between independent data, such as two different intelligence tests.

(3) *Content Validity*, or the consistency of the various individual items which comprise the test. For example, in developing a scale for depression which contains a series of questions, the investigator must evaluate the relationship of each item to the scale score in an experimental situation to determine whether a specific question can make a contribution to the total score. On a depression index, questions related to lowered mood generally have high content validity, while questions about accident proneness will generally have low content validity (although, in a fuller sense, accident proneness may be an indicator of suicidal intent reflecting depressive illness).

(4) *Construct Validity*, or the power of the specific test to measure its underlying concept, its "construct." In clinical situations it is often difficult to relate the "concept" of anxiety to patients' symptoms and behaviors because the concept is elastic and multiform; therefore, to determine construct validity, an investigator must undertake various experiments which involve testing hypotheses about the basic construct. In general, scales and indices of anxiety or depression have limited construct validity because these conditions are conceptually complex.

Reliability

Reliability refers to consistency over a period of time, that is, to a test's capability of producing consistent results when it is administered at different time periods. Of course, intervening variables generally influence the reliability of a psychological test. For example, at a given time a patient may have a high score on a depression index and a few months later, a much lower score for a number of reasons such as changing personal circumstances or treatment. On the other hand, an elderly adult whose life situation is relatively stable and who has only moderate brain damage would be expected to have somewhat similar scores on two tests for organic brain disease administered three months apart.

The scientific value of many psychological tests are dependent upon the norms and standards which have been used for validation and reliability. Importantly, established standards permit comparison of the individual to the group. Patients with physical handicaps cannot be rated scientifically by tests which were standardized on subjects without handicaps. It is also imperative that the examiner use clinical judgments to gauge variations in individual performance. The psychologist's judgments in the testing situation are of tremendous clinical significance when tests are administered to patients from varying ethnic and subcultural backgrounds because many tests are standardized only on homogeneous groups, e.g., white, middle-class students and patients.

FUNCTIONS ASSESSED BY TESTING

Psychological testing generally appraises the patient's intelligence, other intellectual functions, personality characteristics, and symptom patterns for diagnostic and prognostic purposes. For example, what is the patient's intellectual level? Is there evidence of impairment or deterioration? How does the patient utilize his intelligence? Is the patient constricted or does he work up to his potential capacity? How does he approach problem-solving situations: by trial and error? rigidly? confusedly? or antagonistically? Is practical judgment intact? To what degree and under what situations does he show evidence of his ability to conceptualize? Is he an abstract, functional, or concrete thinker? Is memory intact for auditory, visual, rote, meaningful or nonmeaningful material? To what degree is his perceptual organization accurate or distorted?

The affective and conative aspects of the patient's personality structure also emerge during psychodiagnostic testing. For example, testing will reveal the patient's responses to affect-provoking situations, the degree of control that is present, and whether affectivity is expressed or inhibited. Testing will provide evidence about the patient's conation—the striving aspects of his personality which involve motivation and the drive for expression of the self. The psychologist can describe what methods the patient uses to achieve goals and whether these methods are realistic, rigid, spasmodic, or consistent. Are the motivations weak or strong? What are the reactions to stress, conflict, and frustration?

Psychodiagnostic testing can supply vital information about the patient's fantasy life; is it healthy, constructive, passive, regressive or autistic? Also, testing unveils conscious and unconscious concepts of the self, and particularly, the level of self-esteem. Importantly, testing supplies objective data about the patient's capacity for and degree of insight, and his major sentiments, attitudes, drives, basic style of adjustment, conflicts, strengths, and compensations.

In addition to testing the patient formally, the psychologist assesses the patient's behavior and attitude toward the examiner, as well as his attitude toward the tests. Is he hostile, negativistic, compliant, or cooperative? Does he display pleasure, curiosity, apathy, or aversion toward the tests? Does he show differential degrees of interest in the various types of tests? Does he become involved with the testing? Does he give up easily? Does he respond only under urging? What are his reactions to failures or successes during the testing?

TYPES OF TESTS

Some tests are designed to be given to groups; others are presented individually. Group-testing permits large numbers of subjects to be examined simultaneously and is useful in large-scale screening and selection programs in schools, industry, the Armed Forces, etc. Most clinicians prefer the individual approach which allows for more comprehensive observation and greater adaptability in meeting the needs of the patient.

Tests may be verbal or nonverbal. The verbal require the use of language, written or oral, for directions and responses. The nonverbal tests may make use of pictures, symbols, or designs, and are usually paper and pencil type examinations. But when subjects suffer sensory, motor, or language handicaps, the test may be administered with pantomime directions. The more general use of nonverbal tests involves performance tasks employing form boards, blocks, pictures, and other materials in the solution of problems.

Tests of Intellectual Function for Children and Adults

In America, the most widely used tests of intelligence and general ability are the two Wechsler scales: the Wechsler Adult Intelligence Scale (WAIS) and the Wechsler Intelligence Scale for Children (WISC).

The WAIS contains six Verbal and five Performance subscales. The Verbal include tests of Information, Comprehension, Digit-Span, Similarities, Arithmetic, and Vocabulary. The Performance include Picture Arrangement, Picture Completion, Block Design, Object Assembly, and Digit-Symbol tests. The WISC, which is administered to subjects aged five to fifteen is a modified version of the WAIS. A Wechsler scale, the WIPSC is also available for use with preschool children aged three–five.

The mean score for the Wechsler I.Q. is 100; the standard deviations are +15. Fifty percent of the population score between 90-110; 25 percent score below 90 and 25 percent above 110. The lowest 5 percent score below 75 and the highest 5 percent score above 125. Scores between 80-90 are indicative of borderline intelligence, and even lower scores reflect the varying degrees of mental retardation and intellectual deficiencies.

The WAIS reports the subject's separate Verbal and Performance scale scores of intelligence and general ability as well as the Full Scale Score. For a given patient, the Verbal and the Performance scores may differ greatly and this difference may be of clinical significance, particularly when it is fifteen or more points. A significantly lower score on the Verbal than on the Performance scale may be indicative of little formal education, difficulties in the use of English, or the influence of a subcultural background which did not prepare the individal for standardized Verbal intelligence tests. Many such persons will have higher Performance scores than Verbal scores. Sometimes a significantly higher Verbal than Performance score is characteristic for the sociopath who is intrigued when he is engaged in the less tedious Verbal tests, but whose underlying instability is revealed when he is compelled actually to perform or to stick to a task which he may regard as boring, trying, and demanding. A significantly lower Performance than Verbal score, however, may be due to neurologic difficulties, emotional factors such as anxiety, or the individual's capacity to persevere when he is confronted with tasks which require sustained attention and concentration.

The various subtest scores on the WAIS form patterns which can be clinically interpreted. In her book, *Appraising Personality: An Introduction to the Projective Techniques*, Harrower emphasizes that: "There is more to it than the I.Q." For example, she discusses the difference between patients whose scores on the various subtests are relatively consistent and those whose scores on the subtests "scatter" widely. Relatively low scores on a specific subtest may reveal a patient's particular vulnerabilities, for example, difficulty with abstract thinking, anxiety about an unfamiliar task such as arithmetic, or memory difficulties due to organic brain disease. The "scatter" of the scores of the various subtests may be indicative of an erratic performance and thus exemplify a particular patient's behavior problems in real life, or it may, as noted, indicate a specific defect in one or more areas. Harrower describes the clinical information which can be obtained from just the patient's responses. For example, a patient's answers to the Similarities subtest may be a clue to the fact that he sexualizes situations generally, or that he is unable to follow the test instructions because of his own drives, attitudes, or aggressiveness or passivity.

Many psychologists distinguish among abstract, functional, and concrete conceptual approaches. Abstract conceptualizations depend upon an ability to progress beyond immediate sensory stimuli, to delineate and analyze common perceptual properties, to classify forms and categories, and to derive an explanatory principle. The individual with a capacity for abstract conceptualization is also able to keep several aspects of the problem simultaneously in mind, to plan critically, and to shift from one aspect to another. In contrast, the subject who thinks concretely responds to each problem and situation as unique and is unable to remove it from a single class or category. A functional approach categorizes ideas or objects in terms of their utility. Most of the concept-formation tests used are generally qualitative in nature, but the Similarities test in the WAIS can reveal a great deal about the individual's way of thinking and his capacity for abstraction, which, of course, is usually impaired in the patient who is schizophrenic or who has organic brian disease.

Certain cautions in dealing with all tests of Verbal and Performance skills in children should be mentioned. Such tests have primarily two purposes: (1) to determine the present developmental status of the child with respect to the functions being measured at the time of the examination, and (2) to predict intellectual status and future development. The first purpose is satisfied within limits, but predictions about future development are frequently quite dubious. The child may be resistant to the examiner; he may fail to exercise maximum effort; he may be culturally handicapped; or, he may be emotionally upset. Importantly, very small children often show marked fluctuations in the tempo of development. In view of these considerations, care should be exercised in drawing conclusions about young children from test results alone.

In addition to the WIPSC, which is used for preschool children, the Gesell Developmental Schedules are helpful in evaluating children below the age of five. At each age level an inventory of activities is divided into four categories of behavior: (1) Motor, (2) Adaptive, (3) Language, and (4) Personal-Social. Each of these categories of behavior is evaluated by observing the child in a number of standardized situations. Activity is stimulated by presenting the child with various objects, such as a rattle, spoon, cup, form board, etc. In addition, the child's spontaneous activities and locomotion are observed. His performance is recorded by plus and minus signs for each of the items in the four fields mentioned above; standards have been obtained by testing normal children. No precise score is possible in a psychometric sense. The examiner formulates a summarizing statement with a tentative D.Q. (developmental quotient) which is calculated in a manner similar to the I.Q.—by obtaining its ratio to the chronologic age. Such testing does provide a systematic method of observation and analysis of a child's developmental patterns and a differential diagnosis of intelligence in normal, retarded, and superior infants and young children. The testing also is helpful in bringing to light neurologic defects or minor sensory-motor handicaps not revealed by the ordinary modes of examination. Importantly, the testing provides a baseline for systematic follow-up of the very young child's development.

Tests of Intellectual Impairment

The *Bender Visual Motor Gestalt Test* (or Bender-Gestalt) is a simple, widely used test which yields a great deal of information in a short amount of time. The test consists of nine geometric designs, each printed on individual cards. The subject is told that these cards contain figures that the examiner would like him to reproduce on paper. The individual's inability to reproduce the designs or his changes in their configuration is usually evidence of generalized organic brain disease, since the task requires that perception, organizing capacities, and motor skills be intact. The test is interpreted qualitatively; although it does not yield definite scores, it does supply valuable clinical information. For example, an obsessive-compulsive patient may spend a great deal of time meticulously reproducing the rows of dots and other geometric designs; the way that he approaches the task and the constricted exactness of his designs reveal his personality disturbances. Or, a schizophrenic patient may elaborate the simple designs or include extra material which has a highly personalized meaning to him.

The *Object Sorting Test* is now commonly used to evaluate possible impairment of conceptual thinking attributable to brain disease, schizophrenia, etc. The test employs thirty-three familiar objects commonly used in everyday living; for example, pliers, hammer, two nails, two sugar cubes, a real cigar, an imitation cigar, a matchbook, a filing card, a lock, and a bicycle bell. These objects are spread in front of the patient and he has the task of sorting them in different ways. He is directed to select an object and then put together all other objects which he believes can be grouped with his original selection. He may also be told to arrange all the articles into different groups of his own choosing. Or, the examiner may take several groupings and then ask the subject to state a conceptual basis for the arrangement.

Classifications can be made on a concrete basis, according to color, form, or materials (all red objects or all metallic objects); or functionally (hammer and nails); or abstractly (matchbook and a filing card which are similar not only in material but also could be used to start a fire). Often some schizophrenic patients cannot voluntarily make abstract classifications, or their groupings of diverse objects reveal their highly personalized, often bizarre thinking. Patients with generalized severe brain damage often have difficulty arranging the objects unless they can see a simple functional utility for them.

Neuropsychological Tests. The problem of localization of brain damage is an exceedingly complex one because damage in one area often tends to create disturbances in other areas, and also because total functions are the result of integration from many areas; however, neuropsychological testing is useful in evaluating minimal signs of brain damage, particularly in a questionable case. Initial testing provides a baseline for evaluation by subsequent testing and thus may lead to knowledge about diagnosis as well as prognosis. Many individuals whose behavior and mental capacities have appeared unimpaired, have been found during a routine post-mortem examination to have widespread evidence of brain damage. The question then is: to what degree is the altered behavior attributable to organic changes in the central nervous system, and to what degree is it due to psychologic causes? An integrated, comprehensive answer must take into account not only the cerebral impairments, but also the life history, the habitual modes of behavior, stresses and strains, and the physical and biochemical status of the individual.

Aptitude and Vocational Tests

Personality maladjustment may involve an inability to achieve vocational satisfactions, which, in turn, limits the individual's social adaptabilities and exacerbates his difficulties. Guidance in the choice of occupation, therefore, may be of great importance in helping students, young adults, and even persons in mid-life chart courses of study for future vocations. With an adequate appraisal of the individual's educational background, personality characteristics, prime motivations, and intellectual potential as a basis, tests such as the following may be found useful.

Aptitude Tests

An aptitude test is to be distinguished from tests of intelligence, educational achievement, and particular skills or interests. Aptitude tests are designed to tap an individual's potential ability in particular types of specialized activites, ranging from simple sensory and motor performances to extremely complex functions. Tests are available for the assessment of abilities in manual and mechanical dexterity, graphic arts, engineering, and various academic pursuits. The interviewer will often find that consultative work with a Vocational Rehabilitation Counsellor and aptitude testing will benefit psychiatric patients, who, during convalescence are attempting to reorient their lives. Many aptitude tests are available; the choice of the test should take into account the norms for age, sex, and education and the aptitudes to be measured.

Tests of *mechanical aptitude* assess the individual's reaction time, steadiness, speed, and dexterity; various types of jobs require general mechanical ability and even finely differentiated motor skills and coordination. An example of a paper and pencil test in this field is the *Minnesota Paper Form Board Test* which shows two or more parts of a geometric figure correctly assembled, and a series of parts, which, if properly fitted, will also make the correct figure. The subject is required to identify the assembled whole from five choices. This test lends itself to easy objective scoring and measures capacity to visualize and manipulate geometric forms. The *Minnesota Clerical Aptitude Test* and numerous comparable ones evaluate the individual's proficiency in basic skills required in clerical occupations. Tests are also used widely to assess *Professional Aptitudes*, for example, for medicine or law. Aptitude tests can be interpreted only in terms of group norms; therefore, care must be exercised in applying them in an individual case.

Vocational Interests Inventories

These are constructed on the assumption that the effective use of an individual's abilities and aptitudes is dictated by his motivations and interests, i.e., one works best at that which one enjoys the most. The *Kuder Preference Record* is an inventory which includes a large number of items that cover a wide range of activities and proclivities; for example, the subject is asked whether he likes to: "tinker with a broken sewing machine," "play the piano," or "sketch an interesting scene." The inventory is easily scored in terms of percentile ranks in each of a number of areas of vocational interest. These are: outdoor, mechanical, computational, scientific, persuasive, artistic, literary, musical, social service, and clerical. The scores form a profile which shows the individual's high, average, or low percentile ranking on each of the occupational interest-areas. Occupational choices for either single or combined interests are suggested in the manual.

The *Strong Vocational Interests Blank* (SVIB) consists of 400 questions about numerous activities. The items deal with the individual's likes, dislikes, and indifference in categories such as occupations, amusements, and school subjects. In addition to providing indices as to general vocational levels and interests, the SVIB provides ratings for specific occupations.

Such tests indicate avidities rather than specific aptitudes. Therefore, information obtained from aptitude and vocational tests should be collated with other psychological test results, educational records, previous work history, and the general evaluation of personality characteristics. And always, the examiner must use his clinical judgment for interpreting a patient's test results.

Personality Assessment

Two major types of tests are currently employed for personality assessment: (1) the self-report inventories such as the commonly used *Minnesota Multiphasic Personality Inventory* (MMPI) which can be scored objectively, and (2) the projective tests such as the *Rorschach Test* which uses ink blots and the *Thematic Apperception Test* (TAT) which uses pictures to which the individual responds.

The two major types of tests are fundamentally different. The inventories contain lists of questions to which the individual can respond in a limited or specific way, i.e., with a "yes" or "no" answer. Moreover, they are paper and pencil tests or are presented to the individual on plastic cards which he places into the separate "yes"-"no" boxes. The inventories, therefore, involve little or no interaction between the examiner and the subject.

In contrast, the projective techniques contain less structured (TAT) or unstructured (Rorschach) stimuli to which the subject is encouraged to respond as freely and in as many ways as possible. They involve a great deal of interaction between the examiner and the subject. Thus, their use requires that the examiner utilize his clinical skills and abilities for clinical interpretations.

The Minnesota Multiphasic Personality Inventory

The MMPI consists of 566 statements to which the individual being tested is required to give "yes"-"no" answers. His responses yield scores on four validity scales and ten clinical scales. The four validity scales aid the clinician in interpreting the scores on the clinical scales.

The first of the validity scales, the Question (?) scale, is a summation of the items which the subject places in the "cannot say" category. A high score on this scale (300 or more items) makes retesting or the forced answering of neglected items desirable and renders dubious any personality assessment based on the entire test. The second of the validity scales, the Lie (L) scale, consists of items about a number of common human foibles which most persons will admit are true for themselves. Because the statements are "always" or "never" items, a high score on this scale generally indicates that the subject is denying common faults in order to "put himself in a good light." But this scale score should not be used to diagnose "malingering" since it is neither very subtle nor sensitive. The False (F) scale consists of items which are rarely endorsed, such as bizarre or unusual thoughts or actions, peculiar experiences, feelings of isolation, etc. A high score may indicate confusion, an inability to understand the items, random answering, or that the subject is trying to place himself in a "bad light" (cry for help?). The final validity scale, the K scale, provides another measure of the subject's test-taking attitude in that it discriminates between persons trying to make favorable impressions (high scores) and those trying to present spuriously poor pictures of themselves (low scores). It is a more subtle measure of defensiveness than the L scale.

Clinicians generally look at the validity scales in relationship to each other. An F-K index of +7 or more suggests that a person is trying to appear sicker than he is, while an F-K index of −7 or less suggests that he is unwilling to admit to psychological problems.

The ten clinical scales on the MMPI are identified by the names of psychiatric diagnostic categories. However, an elevated score on, for instance, the hysteria or schizophrenia scale, does not imply the presence of typical textbook hysteric or schizophrenic symptoms. Instead, the elevated scale scores and their interrelationships are meaningful only in terms of their dynamic correlates: underlying etiology, interpersonal relations, attitudes toward self and life in general, defensive systems, and general adaptations, rather than psychiatric nosology. Normative values on the validity and clinical scales differ for different populations; for example, college students as a group have much higher than average mean scores on scales K, Pd and Ma, reflecting the usual struggles and uncertainties of their age group. Briefly, the clinical scales may be described as follows:

Hypochrondriasis (Hs). This is a bodily complaint scale, made up of items dealing with concerns about bodily functions and visceral aches and pains. High scorers tend to be sour, pessimistic, complaining, dull. Low scorers may be either capable, physically stable and free of bodily symptoms, or may be denying symptomatology.

Depression (D). The items on this scale deal largely with mood and temperament, tendencies to worry, and expressions of feelings of discouragement with life and plans for the future. High scorers tend to be persons of low morale, easily discouraged, and with a pessimistic outlook; very high D scores may warn of the possibility of suicide. Low scorers are generally alert, cheerful, and extroverted, but sometimes self-seeking and exhibitionistic.

Hysteria (Hy). This scale contains two kinds of items. The first is somewhat similar to the previous scales in that it consist of somatic items, whereas the second deals with "denial" tactics—the refusal to admit any kind of deficiency or maladjustment. High scorers are generally symptomatic, self-centered, manipulative, intolerant of ambivalence in their own feelings, and infantile in their emotional needs, but enthusiastic, uninhibited, and outgoing in their interpersonal contacts. Very low scorers are apt to be misanthropic and asocial.

Psychopathic Deviate (Pd). This scale consists of items concerning social maladjustment and feelings of distance from the group. Boredom and complaints against family are prominent themes. High scorers tend to be outgoing, egocentric, and undependable; often they have not incorporated social and ethical standards. Low scorers tend to be conventional, religious, and overconcerned with social status.

Masculinity-Femininity (Mf). Items on this scale deal with esthetic preferences and interests traditionally associated with masculinity and femininity. High scoring men tend to be passive, imaginative, and sensitive; low scoring men are apt to be easygoing, interested in sports and mechanical activities, and often given to defensive masculinity. High scoring females tend to be confident, aggressive, scientific, and dominating; low scoring females are more likely to be submissive, yielding, constricted, and fault-finding.

Paranoia (Pa). This is gauged by three general classes of items. The first deals with sensitivity to social hurts, the second with excessive moral virtue and denial of suspicion, and the third with suspiciousness and complaint of persecution. High scorers are described as rigid, hard to convince, suspicious, and brooding. Low scorers tend to be evasive and stubborn.

Psychasthenia (Pt). The items on this scale deal with narcissistic preoccupations, magical thinking, sado-masochistic tendencies, phobic and compulsive behavior, and vague feelings of influence. High scorers tend to be tense, insecure, indecisive and unable to concentrate. Low scorers are usually relaxed, easygoing, confident.

Schizophrenia (Sc). The items in this scale are based upon responses made by patients who exhibit delusions, hallucinations and bizarre behavior. They deal with somatic symptoms, peculiar bodily dysfunctions, and feelings of alienation, dissatisfaction, and depression. High scorers feel remote and unloved and show tendencies toward secretiveness and strongly autistic fantasies.

Hypomania (Ma). This scale contains items dealing with expansiveness and egotism, irritability, amorality, and feelings of euphoria. High scorers tend to be warm, expansive, and outgoing, but sometimes emotionally unstable, tense, and hyperactive. Low scorers tend to be listless, apathetic, and show lack of drive or ambition.

Social Introversion-Extraversion (Si). This scale deals with social participation and emotional expression. High scorers are generally shy, quiet, and retiring. Low scorers are considered to be sociable, active, and outgoing. Thus, an individual's score places him on an introversion-extroversion continuum.

Clinical Interpetation of the MMPI

Each of the ten clinical scales on the MMPI yields a score which is plotted on the Profile Sheet. High or low scores on any of the individual scales can be easily detected since the Profile Sheet indicates the "normal" range. Since the MMPI has been standardized with very large groups and subgroups of the general population, as well as with psychiatric and medical patients, the Profile has obvious clinical value. Moreover, during the last ten years computerized interpretation, systems have been developed and are being modified and refined to enhance their validity and clinical utility. A recent review* of "Computers in Psychiatry" stated that "no other test is likely to overtake the MMPI for many years." A massive amount of research is going into the refinement of the computerized interpretation systems.

Although many workers have attempted to give clinical interpretations to a high score on just one of the clinical scales, it is generally unwise to attempt to use an MMPI subscale score as a measure of psychiatric diagnosis. The Hypomania (Ma) scale, for example, does not diagnose manic-depressive illness, although it gives some information about the individual's self-report of his sociability and activity. The Pyschasthenia (Pt) scale measures anxiety and tension, but a high score on the scale is not pathogonomic of an anxiety state. The greatest value of the MMPI lies in the overall configuration of the patient's scores on the various scales and the patterns which disclose information about his personality.

In clinical practice, therefore, the interrelationships between the various scale scores are usually much more important than a single high score. Patients with many bodily complaints tend to score high on the Hs, the Hy,

* Psychiatric Annals, December, 1972, is devoted exclusively to the use of computers in psychiatry and deals extensively with the computerized interpretations of the MMPI.

and the D scales. Most mental patients score high on both the D scale and
the Pt scale since depression and anxiety are fundamental complaints. It is
difficult to evaluate psychosis from the MMPI Profile, but high scores on
the Pa and Sc scales should alert the clinician to the possibility that the
patient is psychotic. The computerized interpretations describe various
syndromes and also list a number of critical items which may be indicative
of serious symptomatology and which warrant clinical evaluation.

Although the MMPI was originally devised as an aid for psychiatric
diagnosis—for separating normals from patients and for differential diagnosis—it is most useful as a screening procedure, particularly since the
development of the computerized interpretations and the increasing use of
the test with patients in diverse settings. However, any individual patient's
scores must be evaluated in the light of the information obtained during the
psychiatric interview.*

Projective Techniques

The term *projection* refers in a general way to the human tendency to
try to understand strange concepts in familiar terms and to identify and
interpret them according to a personal system of values. Thus, the more
ambiguous, the more unfamiliar, and the more unstructured the stimulus,
the more the individual will be forced to "round out" or complete the perceptual experience in terms of his own ideas. Confronted with a strange
and amorphous ink blot, he will be compelled to rely more on his own
inventiveness and ingenuity in responding to the stimulus than if he had
only to respond "yes" or "no" to a question on an inventory. Because the
projective techniques can reveal the individual's highly personalized way of
perceiving and integrating unfamiliar stimuli, and thus tap his emotional
tensions, the interpretation of the responses requires great skill on the part
of the examiner. From his knowledge of personality variables and functions
and from his familiarity in dealing with projective data, the psychologist
can make inferences about the subject's motivations, attitudes, wishes,
fantasies, ways of handling interpersonal situations, and value systems.

The Sentence Completion Test

In this test the subject is asked to complete a sentence after the examiner provides one or more words verbally or on printed forms. Usually the
test is made up of fifty items or more, tapping a number of areas in which
the examiner would like to discover the subject's relatively conscious atti-

* *The Physician's Guide to the MMPI*, by Patricia King-Ellison Good and John P. Brantner, offers a succinct description of the MMPI and its use in clinical settings.

tudes and predispositions. There are many sentence completion tests currently available, but the usual way of presenting the sentence is in the third person ("Mary was happiest when _____." "He loved his mother, but _____."). Consciously acceptable attitudes are more apt to be revealed by the first person approach, whereas the third person form may disclose rejected personal qualities.

Since the purpose of the method is to sound out the attitudes in a variety of areas and to provide the examiner with a general picture or characterologic portrait of the subject, some examiners make up their own test forms to fit the individual or to tap areas in which they do not have much information. The sentence completion forms on the market are generally structured to investigate certain large areas of personality functioning: e.g., attitudes toward parents, peers, superiors or authority figures, self, or sex, and verbalizations about ambitions, wishes, happiest memories, private frustrations, and other topics.

The Thematic Apperception Test

The Thematic Apperception Test (TAT) is made up of a number of cards presenting achromatic illustrations of people in some sort of interaction or situation. For example, Card 1 shows a small boy sitting at a table with a violin before him; Card 10 shows an elderly man and woman embracing; Card 16 is a blank card upon which the subject is asked to visualize and picture what he likes. Certain of the cards are designed for use only with men, women, boys, or girls. The subject is asked to "make up a story about this picture" and to include all the important elements: what led up to the scene in the picture, what is going on, and how it will turn out. Additional encouragement or direction is sometimes given in the form of subsidiary questions: What are the people feeling and thinking? What relationships do they have, one to another? What other people (not shown) play a part in the story? As may be seen, the fantasies so elicited are derived from conscious and unconscious attitudes about important people and situations in the subject's life, his basic interpersonal values, and his anxieties, social weaknesses, prejudices, hatreds, loves, and the ways in which he implements his major goals.

*Use of TAT as Mental Status Data.** To Card 4 (a picture of a man in the foreground experiencing some emotional reaction, and a woman slightly in the background, reaching her arms out toward him, both are facing forward—looking out of the picture) a male subject supplied the following story:

* Cf. Masserman, J. and Balken, Eve.

"Oh. This looks like a scene you'd see in a movie. Looks like a rough—not rough—shady character. This man's tearing away from this woman. She could be the sweet type, trying to make him a home—or maybe the sly type! But he's tearing away . . . hate in his eyes. They're not living in a very good place . . . there's a calendar on the wall. But it looks like he's setting out on a mission—or maybe he's running away. And the woman is running away—trying to keep him there. She seems very sweet, doesn't look like the sly type, although she could be slipping him a Mickey or something. Maybe she's his wife, although I don't see a ring on her third finger, so she couldn't be his wife. (Examiner: 'How does it turn out?') If I myself were that man, I'd stay. But I think he'll leave . . . "

Further questioning by the examiner could have elicited more information: Why would the man run away? What was driving him away? What was the actual relationship between the man and the woman? Why was he angry? What was *she* thinking and feeling? And many others. But the fact that the subject avoided these critical areas becomes highly important; as a result of these neglects, his story becomes interpersonally impoverished.

Further attempts to neutralize the emotion-filled scene appeared in many ways. The situation is a "scene . . . in a movie"; the woman is either the sweet "type" or the sly "type." The man is alternately hero and villain. The story-people's motivations become strangely variable. He is at once hating, running away, on a mission, leaving. He is initially a "rough, shady character," but later being victimized ("slipping him a Mickey"). She is "trying to make him a home," "trying to keep him there" (against his will), "seems very sweet." The possible marital relationship is dismissed on a technicality.

In a few short, halting sentences, a picture of the subject's interpersonal attitudes, ways of dealing with social situations, sense of values, ambivalences, interpersonal feelings, and approach to problems is revealed as his fantasies come tumbling out. By setting up, rejecting, modifying, and augmenting repeated hypotheses, the examiner can develop a rounded out picture of a major portion of the subject's personality structure.

To complete the TAT, the psychologist writes a summary of the important materials gleaned from the subject's story productions. The manner in which the test is actually interpreted and translated into a picture of specific personality operations rests upon a number of assumptions and hypotheses about fantasy productitns in general and about the TAT pictures as stimulus materials in particular.

Interpretation of the Fantasy Material. Morgan and Murray (1935) interpret the patient's fantasies as expressive of personalized "needs" or "drives" which are opposed to external forces of an inanimate or social nature. The interaction of specific needs and presses then constitutes "themata" into which the fantasies may be analyzed according to a standard schedule. From a less formalized standpoint, however, the rationale of the test may be regarded as based on the "projective" dynamisms of all fantasy formations. Essentially, the patient reacts to the relatively neutral stimuli of the test pictures (a) peopling his fantasies with *dramatis personae* who represent important influences in his own life, (b) placing these imaginary personages in situations that symbolize his own conscious or unconscious conflicts, and (c) resolving these conflicts in ways indicative of the solutions he seeks for his own difficulties (Masserman and Balken). In most cases the patient does not recognize these relatively direct relationships; for this reason, or with the defensive rationalization that he is "talking only about imaginary people," he may imbue his fantasies with relative freedom of symbolization and movement, and so disclose significant anamnestic and dynamic material not otherwise easily obtained. An example illustrates the point:

CASE 21.   Anamnestic use of TAT fantasy material. A middle-aged woman was admitted with severe depressive and anxiety symptoms which, she insisted, could have no relationship to her life situation and must therefore be due to organic disease. History-taking, even under Amytal hypnosis, furnished little additional information. In response to pictures F17, N2 and F14, however, she produced the following fantasies:

F17: (A girl grasping the shoulders of an elderly woman on a step below her): "At first glance you might think this was one woman trying to see another woman's tonsils. But no. She is showing the proper technique of how to strangle... your landlady. One never knows when this will happen in the best of families....It's well to have a stairway so that a fall might finish the job."

N2: (A woman looks at a reclining man): "It might be a landlady finding a dead body... of a roomer... a suicide."

F14: (A girl holding a man away with one arm): "John was a dentist... Betty needed dental work and came to him....She was pretty and smart looking. After the appointment, John, who was slightly erotic, made an unpleasant proposition to Betty. She is still holding him at arm's length because he hasn't enough money and cannot furnish enough security to make it interesting."

Later, when the content of her TAT was recalled in an interview, the patient revealed that her life had recently been made miserable by a preemptive mother-in-law (the landlady) and that semiconscious murderous impulses had caused reactions of severe anxiety, fears of punishment and thoughts of suicide. In hostile jealousy of her husband, moreover, she had conducted a flirtation with a retired physician but had resisted his sexual advances.

Certain characteristics of fantasies are usually significant. For instance, there may be almost unmistakable references to the transference relationship between the physician and the patient: e.g., the former may be embodied in the character of a wise teacher or a kind priest, or variously condemned in the person of a tyrannical father, a neglected nurse or a ruthless detective. Similarly, suspicions, fears, hostilities, aggressions and various combinations of attitudes may pervade the fantasies, or their symbolic material may indicate narcissistic, oral, anal, fetishistic, or homosexual fixations. Finally, as the patient's therapy progresses, significant changes in his associations to the same pictures occur on retest and so furnish indices of exacerbation or resolution of the patient's intrapsychic conflicts. Masserman and Balken (1949) concluded:

"From a psychoanalytic standpoint many of the phantasies reveal in symbolic form the intrapsychic urges, desires, repressions and conflicts of the patient and thus indicate the unconscious determinants of his neurosis or psychosis. In the same way, the phantasies frequently provide an index of the status of the patient's transference, his reaction to the therapeutic situation and the depth or superficiality of his subsequent emotional reintegrations, although, because of various complicating factors, these interpretations cannot be validly made in all cases.

"From a psychiatric standpoint, the phantasies are sometimes of aid in securing a significant anamnesis and in emphasizing certain salient clinical features of the case. In certain instances the phantasies also help to orient the psychotherapy and the environmental readjustments of the patient."

"Diagnostic" Significance of the Fantasies. The patient's fantasies are meaningful in the following respects:

"Intelligence": The fantasies of mentally deficient patients show poverty of ideational material, lack of categorical meaning, naiveté in dramatic structure, and general dearth of originality and force. In contrast, patients of superior intelligence, when not neurotically inhibited, produce fantasies rich in detail, delightfully versatile, and charged with creative invention.

"Anxiety states": Patients with marked free-floating anxiety are, in general, hesitant, guarded and noncommital in their associations unless or until a trustful rapport has been established with the examiner. When this occurs, however, their fantasies become peopled by boldly drawn protagonists who, placed in moving, dramatic situations of conflict, act in ways that are generally futile and tragic. Severely anxious patients may then identify themselves directly with these characters and thus give their stories a frankly autobiographic cast.

"Conversion reactions": In contrast, in patients in whom manifest anxiety has been largely alleviated by symptom formation and passive regression, the fantasies become easy, flippant, superficially erotic, and may even involve persons identifiable as members of the subject's immediate family —although in this case the erotic scenes generally end frustratingly. Fixed hypochondriacal tendencies are often projected onto a martyred, misunderstood, long-suffering hero in each of the stories.

"Obsessive-compulsive neuroses": The ambivalence that underlies compulsive and phobic reactions may be reflected in the patient's fantasies, as already indicated, by a pervading uncertainty and querulous indecision in which he may even appeal to the examiner for help in bringing the detailed, fruitless stories to some conclusion. Thematic fears appear repeatedly, sometimes in a setting of wishfully charged fascination with the situation obsessively feared. In compensation, the hero of the fantasy is often pictured as a being who, though superior in intelligence, courage, righteousness and other excellent qualities, cannot cope with an illogical, contentious and uncertain environment.

"Depression": The fantasies of depressed patients are characteristically retarded, halting, fragmented, produced under a pall of discouragement and with a sense of intense effort. In addition, they are usually preoccupied with guilt, self-depreciation and nihilistic futility, beneath which lie pathetic or covertly hostile and imperative appeals for protection and succor.

"Paranoia": As could be expected, the productions of paranoid patients are often deliberately evasive and sometimes contain specific misinterpretations of the motives of the examiner and the purposes of the test. Highly circumlocutory and symbolic readings of the cards may be given, although occasionally pictures suggestive of homosexual relationships produce anxiety reactions approaching disruptive panic.

"Schizophrenia": Marked schizophrenic self-isolation is indicated by bizarre characterizations, interpenetrations of time, space and personal movement, and highly abstract themata in baroque and startlingly fantastic productions with little evident relationship to the stimulus picture. With greater impoverishment of interest, transference, and verbalization, the responses deteriorate to offhand dismissals of the pictures and fragmented or verbigerated descriptions or even negativistic gestures or complete mutism. (Masserman and Balken, 1949.)

The Word-Association Test

This technique involves presenting to the subject, either orally or graphically, a list of words to which he is asked to respond with "the first thing that comes to mind." Mixed in with "neutral" commonplace words are usually others intended to elicit associations and reactions to charged topics which disclose certain aspects of the personality. Clues to the subject's personality are obtained in three major ways: (1) by analyzing responses or associations to words on which he shows some "emotional arousal"; (2) by noting the occurrence of blockings or hesitations; and (3) by evaluating the conformity or uniqueness of a subject's responses as compared to norms for his culture or diagnostic group. The element of time-to-react is an important factor since it frequently elicits blocking or reveals intensity of affect. Other qualities are of secondary interpretative significance, but the test can reveal perseveration of responses, clang associations, object-naming of things in the testing situation, self-references, multiple word reactions and other evidence of associative disturbances.

There are various standard word-association forms available (e.g. the Kent-Rosanoff), but many examiners prefer to develop their own lists to conform to specific needs for information. Variations of the technique in which multiple choice responses are presented to the subject along with the stimulus word, or in which the subject is requested to associate in sequence to the responses set off by an initial stimulus word, are of some use for special cases.

The Rorschach Technique

The Rorschach is probably the best known and most extensively used of the projective techniques. It is a method used to describe personality in terms of dynamic processes and is thought, more or less generally, to be particularly sensitive in revealing "deeper, unconscious layers" of psychologic operations. Klopfer has listed seven major areas about which the Rorschach gives information:

(1) The degree and mode of control with which the subject tries to regulate his experiences and actions.

(2) The "responsiveness of his energies" to stimulations from outside and "promptings from within."

(3) His approach to given problems and situations.

(4) His creative or imaginative capacities, and the use he makes of them.

(5) An evaluation of the subject's degree of security or anxiety.

(6) A general estimate of intellectual level and the major qualitative features of the subject's thinking.

(7) The relative degree of maturity in his total personality development.

As originally designed by Hermann Rorschach and elaborated by Klopfer, Beck, Harrower, and others, the test consists of ten cards on each of which is printed a roughly symmetrical inkblot. Five are achromatic and five are in various colors. The cards are presented to the subject in sequence and he is asked to report what the blots suggest to him. The examiner records verbatim responses, time per response and per card, card turning, and other pertinent behavioral data. After the last card has been returned, the examiner and the subject go back over the responses, one by one, in order to determine more exactly the nature of the associations. This aids the examiner in deciding how to score the individual responses.

Scoring usually involves marking down symbols to represent three major categories of information about the specific responses. The first category is LOCATION, i.e., whether all or only part of the blot is used in a particular response, the relative *size* of the detail used, and the *area* of the blot in which is falls. The second category is DETERMINANT, i.e., what determines the character of the response: form alone, form combined in some manner with the color or shading of the blot, color or shading alone, movement impressions in the blot, etc. If form plays an important part in the response, the examiner determines how "accurate" or appropriate the response is to the "actual" shape of the blot. To determine the appropriateness of responses he may refer to the available statistical tables, or rely on his own judgment. The final category is CONTENT, i.e., the denotation of the general class of objects into which the response falls: A for animal; H for human; Na for nature, etc. The examiner may also note additional scoring symbols, such as the *popularity* (or conformity) of the response, unusual movement qualities (inanimate or animal movement), *tendencies* toward the use of a particular determinant, or the form-organization scores (cf. Beck).

Once the scoring is completed, the examiner fills in a test protocol or Summary Sheet, on which all symbols of a particular class are totaled. He may also compute certain ratios involving various scoring symbols which many examiners have found useful. Then the task of interpreting the material is at hand.

Interpretation of the Rorschach

Like all samples of behavior, the Rorschach Technique may be approached in interpretation from many directions. The examiner may begin with the protocol or Summary Sheet and proceed through the test, response by response, vicariously experiencing and interpreting the subject's handling of the perceptual task. Or he may score the responses in categories—location, determinant and content—and observe how each of these dimensions is affected by the appearance of a new card, a traumatic association, etc. However, in every approach the examiner must apply to Rorschach interpretation the basic principles of a dynamic theory of personality. In addition, there are several secondary assumptions:

Most subjects feel that *what* they see in the blots is the critical material, whereas, in actuality, it is the *way* in which the blots are seen that is most significant. The first two of the three scoring categories—location and determinant—indicate the subject's approach. Thus, the location category refers not only to *where* a particular association is seen, but also to its general size—whether the association includes all of the blot, an important portion of the blot, or a relatively minor portion. Such information can reveal how a subject characteristically approaches new situations—e.g., whether he prefers to analyze a situation cautiously, bit by bit, or quickly dispense with it by grasping at its most obvious components. The location category, along with the number of responses a subject produces, yields a rough index of how he surveys his world and what intellectual resources he brings to bear in handling it. An additional scoring symbol (S), standing for White Space when the subject associates to a blank portion of the care or an empty spot in the blot, is usually scored with location.

The largest fund of information about the way in which a subject sees the blots comes from the determinant category. Many of the ways that a subject perceives and integrates the blots have been isolated. Some of the major ones are: the use of color, the use of black or white as color, the shading nuances, the perception of movement in the blots, and the three-dimensional responses.

When a subject uses *color* to identify a response, it is usually in combination with some form. A subject may see not only "a bird"—he may see "a *red* bird." He may also see green grass, in which case the color seems to be more important than the form it takes. Or he may see an explosion, a response to which form contributes little, whereas color contributes almost wholly. The use of color, not only in Rorschach but also in advertising and art, is generally thought to evoke "feeling" as expressed in perceptiveness form, and control. The spontaneous *explosion* response, however, suggests a loss of control since it is relatively formless and thoughtless.

In general, the frequency with which the subject uses color responses is merely a rough quantitative measure suggesting the degree to which he will relate affectively to his environment. The character of the relationship is something else again, i.e., the color red can symbolize warmth to one subject or anger to another. These differentiations can be determined only by examining the individual responses in which color is used. When the subject uses the blackness or whiteness on the blot or card as color (a black dog, a white snowman), the responses are interpretable in the same manner as those which involve colors.

A preoccupation with blank portions of the card (white spaces) may have a special meaning. For example, identifying these spaces as *white only* is, in fact, a refusal, neglect or failure to follow the test instructions; instead of seeing something in *the blot, the subject is using the places where there is no* blot. In addition, this is a true reversal of figure and ground in the perceptual task set by the Rorschach. The interpretation of white space responses follows naturally from these observations; in effect, the subject is exercising a kind of self-assertiveness, if not negativism, in the way he is relating to the task and the world.

The *shading responses* have been one of the most investigated of all Rorschach determinants. To quote Klopfer, "shading responses are those where the subject uses the darker and lighter shading of the gray areas, and occasionally also that of the chromatic areas, to contribute to one of the three following effects."

(1) Shading gives the impression of surface or texture ("it looks like a fur rug; I can run my hand over the card and almost feel the texture").

(2) Shading gives the impression of three dimensions or depth, either in the sense of diffusion ("A mist—a gray, cloud-like mist") or vista ("A town, way off in the distance").

(3) Shading gives the impression of a three-dimensional expanse projected on a two-dimensional plane ("A portion of the blot seems to stick right up, like a plateau").

Rorschach studies indicate that all use of shading reveals the way in which a person thinks and feels about himself. Since the factor of form combines with the shading responses as it did with color, the multiple variations in feeling tones can be ascertained with unusual sensitivity. Some investigators also believe that surface or texture responses reveal "nurturant" needs on the part of the subject to make "contact" with sources of gratification directly and concretely. The other two major types of shading responses are also related to the way in which the subject handles his needs for affection, security, belongingness and importance. For example, extensive use of vista responses ("a town in the distance," "a man up on a cliff") suggests a feeling of loneliness, of isolation, or of distance in relation to the subject's expectations of gratification from his environment. His absorption in the formless, diffuse shading qualities of a blot strongly implies the presence of painful anxiety.

The use of shading in conjunction with color is a not infrequent occurrence in Rorschach examinations. Depending on the interaction and use of these two determinants, they may indicate intense ambivalence or guilt; conversely, the subtle use of shadings in color or tones of color may reveal the presence of tact, gentleness and confidence in relating to other people.

When a subject reports *movement* (M) in an association to an inkblot ("a man running," "a woman talking") he is doing something perceptually unique in the sense that he *adds more to the blot* than in the case of any other determinant. It is true that some areas of some blots tend to elicit more M responses than others but in every case the subject supplies the concrete qualities of muscular tension and activity. The employment of movement in a response also carries with it empathic or sympathic dynamisms and fantasies. These include the ability to delay action, to think through situations and predict outcomes, to enjoy gratification vicariously and symbolically, and to experience in imagery that which would be difficult or dangerous to experience behaviorally. In addition, the use of M denotes those areas of activity in which he feels he must enjoy fantasied rather than direct gratifications.

Motion is also seen in many other objects besides human beings. Inanimate, animal, and human movements are on a continuum, expressive of specific or general areas of developmental conflict. Inanimate movement represents the attempts of the subject to deal with early infantile security operations at a time in his life when all pressures on him came through the medium of vague but insistent physical forces. Animal movement seems more directly related to the development of the spontaneous, unbridled activity in childhood, when the subject exulted in the powers of his own body and enjoyed his most satisfying relationships with animals and objects. Human movement responses deal with the more recent experiences of adolescence and adulthood when the greatest experiences and tests are in the field of interpersonal relations and when the capacity for fantasy undergoes its most subtle changes and develops its complex matrix of values, internalizations, empathies and maneuvers.

In addition to the interpretation of the single or complex determinants of the Rorschach associations, many investigators also employ certain ratios which have been developed over a number of years. The most widely used, perhaps, is the M/C ratio, comprising the total number of movement responses over a summation of color values. This ratio is roughly indicative of the direction of the subject's conative investments, whether he is more introspective (overbalanced toward M) or more responsive toward the environment (overbalanced toward C). Another ratio frequently employed is the W/M ratio, in which W stands for the *total number* of responses to the blot as a whole and M stands for total number of movement responses. When W greatly exceeds M, the subject may be a person who rushes impulsively into things without much consideration of the consequences. When the ratio is overbalanced toward M, the subject is likely to be cautious, thoughtful and to prefer rumination to action. A third important ratio is the number of *good* form responses over the total number of form responses. This yields a percentage which has been demonstrated to be roughly correlated with what can be described as integrative capacity or "ego strength." Other Rorschach ratios or indices are of lesser clinical importance.

The Rorschach Technique has two major advantages in producing a picture of personality operations. First, its ambiguous stimuli (inkblots) allow for the greatest expression of individuality on the part of the subject. Second, its interpretation emphasizes a holistic description of the personality. It is obvious that each new clue found on a Rorschach production in some way affects the entire personality picture. And it is precisely because of these two qualities that more skill and experience is demanded of the Rorschach interpreter than is the case with any other psychologic procedure.

Clinical Interpretation of the Rorschach. In her discussion of the Rorschach Technique, Harrower emphasizes that perception and action are intimately connected and that: "The different worlds as experienced by different individuals lead to behavior which is appropriate for the world as they experience it. Thus we are justified in making some predictions about behavior from what the patient sees. Conversely, where the behavioral pattern is well-known, we may catch a glimpse through the ink blot worlds of the *types of distorted experiences* which are giving rise to disturbed behavior."

The Rorschach, therefore, can reveal a great deal of important clinical material. Highly anxious patients, for example, may display aversion to the unfamiliar stimulus of the ink blot, or may block when they are presented with a color card. Their defenses against anxiety show up when they begin to respond carefully and haltingly as they attempt to constrict the stimulus. Depressed patients ordinarily give only a few responses and often respond mainly to the darker, sombre portions of the ink blot.

Obsessively compulsive patients may boringly work with the minor or small areas of shading and give multiple responses to a single card as they endeavor to give meaning to bits and pieces of the ink blot. Patients' sexual disturbances are evidenced by their seeing genitalia or sexual activity in numerous ink blots, or, conversely, by denying that any of the stimuli (particularly Card 6) suggest the genitalia. The schizophrenic patients' reactions to the Rorschach cards indicate their difficulties with boundaries, and thus reality. Often, these patients' bizarre, highly personalized responses are indicative of the diagnosis. Brain-damaged persons may not be able to respond to the amorphus stimuli of the ink blot at all. Or they may give a very limited number of responses, repeating over and over again "it's an animal," thus indicating by their concrete responses that the capacity for abstract thinking is impaired.

The Figure-Drawing Test

For some time, art productions have been used as a source of projective materials with highly gratifying results. The analysis of paintings, drawings or designs produced from mosaic pieces has played an important part in the examination and treatment of children. The use of these materials with adults has been less extensive but equally gratifying.

The method of obtaining a figure drawing is simple: The subject is presented with paper and pencil and asked to draw the figure of a person. In some cases, he is then asked to draw the figure of a person of the opposite sex. The simplicity of the task should not obscure its effectiveness in motivating a subject to produce significant material. Drawing human figures is a favorite occupation during the child's formative period and is an important means of communication and expression at an age when speech is not so facile a mode of expression as in adulthood. The actual completion of the task requires fewer coordinative movements than the writing of one's name.

Many authorities, notably Schilder, have written extensively on the significance of the body image as the medium for the expression of needs, attitudes, perceptual configuration, etc. When a subject sets out to draw a human figure, he must fall back on the images of himself and of other people he has known and seen. The picture he produces naturally becomes composite by virtue of his selective facility in terms of his own experience, identifications, defenses and projections. Thus, many sources are tapped in the production of a human figure. Cultural or sociological forces influence the kind or type of human to be drawn. Body shape, age, sex, and function are obviously important determinants in orienting and relating to the milieu.

The part or parts of the body emphasized in the drawings become significant; they reveal the person's own need-systems and meaningful contacts with the environment. For example, emphasis in the drawing of the mouth region by patients with oral problems is a commonplace observation, whereas patients suffering from auditory hallucinations have been found to draw ornate and complex ear structures on their figures. The quality of the body "boundaries" may be indicative of how distinct the subject sees himself in relation to other people and things. In addition to these dynamic dimensions in the interpretation of figure drawings, the more formal qualities of the drawing are significant. The size of drawing is most obvious, but placement on the page, quality of the lines (sketched or solid and hard), erasures, the position of the figure (profile or front view, motionless or active), the detail of the drawing, and the time required for the drawing are other important factors.

As with most other projective methods, the examiner's skill in interpreting the productions is the most important factor in determining the value of the technique. In addition to a thorough understanding of personality dynamics, the examiner must have a wide experience with a large number of drawings by a variety of subjects about whom adequate supplementary information is available.

INDICATIONS FOR PSYCHOLOGICAL TESTING

Assessment of Mental Functions

Since 1905, when Binet developed his classic intelligence scale, psychological tests have been used for screening school children and determining an individual's intellectual potential. The Wechsler Adult Intelligence Scale (the WAIS) and the Wechsler Intelligence Scale for Children (the WISC) are particularly useful for diagnosing mental retardation in adults or children. Furthermore, the psychiatric interviewer can use the WAIS to determine whether a subject has borderline intelligence and thus differentiate from a patient with an inadequate personality or one who may be an ambulant schizophrenic. The numerous individuals with low normal or borderline intelligence are seriously handicapped in our modern world. Previously, many of them could live satisfying lives in a rural environment or a simple urban setting, but with the complexities of modern technology throughout our society, such individuals are in a relatively worse predicament than in the past. Increasingly, they are confronted by bewildering situations and subjected to the massive overstimulation of modern life. As a result, they manifest emotional distress and neurotic disorders which can be accurately diagnosed and treated most effectively when it is understood that their intellectual capacities are limited.

Psychodiagnostic testing is especially important in the evaluation of children with birth injuries or sequelae of central nervous system diseases; the psychological evaluation aids materially in planning educational and therapeutic programs. When working with adolescents and young adults, the psychiatric interviewer needs to know about the young patient's intellectual abilities to fulfill his vocational ambitions. Some college students, who present neurotic complaints, have elected courses of study beyond their capabilities. When the interviewer has an accurate appraisal of such a patient's intellectual potential he can guide him into a field which is less stressful and hopefully more healthful.

Patients with organic brain disease usually show some impairment of their intellectual functions. These should be measured by psychological testing to determine the extent of the damage, and also to provide a baseline for gauging subsequent evaluations and the rate of deterioration. In addition to intelligence, psychodiagnostic testing will also provide significant information about a patient's capacities for memory and more subtle aspects of organic brain disease such as diminished powers for abstraction and flawed judgment.

Differential Diagnosis

Although the interviewer will find that he can directly diagnose various psychiatric disorders more quickly and more precisely as he gains experience, supplementary psychological testing is a valuable diagnostic procedure for a number of reasons: (1) it has educational benefits for the interviewer; (2) there may be a time pressure for diagnosis; (3) when litigation is involved, the test scores and other data from psychodiagnostic testing are regarded as more tangible than clinical impressions; and, (4) for all interviewers, regardless of experience, testing supports or rejects hypotheses, and even when there is a marked difference between the clinical impressions and the results of testing, this difference, in itself, should require further assessment.

Conflicts and Mental Mechanisms

For some greatly repressed neurotics, fundamental conflicts may be revealed more quickly by projective testing than by a number of hours of interviewing. For example, deep-seated conflicts about sexuality may be unveiled by the patient's responses to the Rorschach cards; or, the responses to the color in the cards may betray an aversion to blood that is indicative of a serious fear of death. The MMPI contains the Welsh Anxiety and Repression Scales; the low anxiety and high repression scores of the typical "hysteric" indicate the extent of repression, and, conversely, very low repression scores may exemplify the schizophrenic's relatively deficient use of repression. The extensive use of denial, and particularly projection, will generally be manifested by the patient's responses to projective tests and thus reveal serious distortions of reality often attributable to psychosis.

Projective tests such as the Rorschach and the TAT provide valuable information about the patient's sexual identification. The Mf (masculine-feminine) subscale score on the MMPI also indicates fundamental personality traits which may or may not be congruent with the patient's gender.

Convalescence and Prognosis

For patients with physical or psychologic disorders, or admixtures thereof, serial testing will provide an accurate index of the patient's progress. Moreover, tests indicate what tasks the patient can perform and thus be helpful in developing convalescent programs. When, for example, the physically ill patient with some degree of organic brain disease is presented with occupational therapy tasks which exceed his capabilities, he is likely to regress or become depressed because of his failures. Conversely, a patient's convalescent program can be retarded when his prescribed activites are uninteresting and far below his capabilities.

A psychiatrically ill patient's prognosis cannot be assessed from the results of psychological testing when he first becomes ill or when he is acutely disturbed. But serial testing over the period of time supplies further data for prognosis. Generally, when a patient's psychological test results show no improvement over the course of a year, the prognosis can be considered as guarded. The results of the tests, however, must always be placed in the specific context and considered as one part of the total diagnostic and prognostic evaluation.

Special Indications*

Special indications for psychodiagnostic testing are related primarily to cases in which litigation is now or is potentially involved. These include: (1) patients with posttraumatic or compensation neurosis, (2) competency cases, particularly patients with organic brain syndromes, (3) cases involving divorce, custody, or wills, in which the interviewer will have to testify in court, and (4) in all instances in which the interviewer is a court-appointed witness—particularly in criminal cases.

Strengths and Weaknesses

Too often psychodiagnostic testing is used primarily to reveal deviancy; however, the highly developed battery of tests administered by the clinical psychologist can also explicate the patient's strengths as well as his deficiencies or manifestations of illness. The strengths include special talents and personality characteristics on which the patient can build a more satisfying life.

REFERRAL FOR PSYCHODIAGNOSTIC TESTING

When the interviewer refers a patient for psychodiagnostic testing he should supply the psychologist with the reasons for the referral and the

* Cf. Schwab, *Handbook of Psychiatric Consultation* and Wortis and Halpern, *Medical Clinics of North America.*

essential facts about the patient's complaints, psychosocial stresses, and physical illnesses which may coexist. In the past, some clinical psychologists were very willing to test patients using blinded procedures, i.e., all clinical information was withheld from the psychologist who then relied exclusively on the results of the tests. Such excessive emphasis on objectivity was useful as an experimental approach for validating tests, but is also highly artificial and certainly not always in the patient's best interests. Therefore, the psychiatric interviewer should summarize the relevant clinical data on the written request for testing and, whenever possible, personally apprise the psychologist about the clinical considerations as fully as possible.

In addition to basic data referring to mental and physical illnesses, the psychiatric interviewer should state clearly the questions which he wishes the psychologist to answer from the testing. These questions may pertain to differential diagnosis or request confirmation of a specific diagnosis, but the entire psychodiagnostic testing procedure can supply much more valuable information about the patient when the interviewer *also* asks specifically about the patient's conflicts, psychodynamics, and particularly, his strengths and weaknesses.

When the psychologist is supplied with this much information and is aware of the interviewer's hypotheses, as well as his particular concerns about a given case, the data from the testing achieve their greatest value as they are incorporated into a comprehensive diagnostic, prognostic and therapeutic formulation.

REFERENCES

1. Allen, R. M.: *Student's Rorschach Manual.* New York, International Universities Press, 1966.
2. Balken, E. R. and Masserman, J. H.: The language of phantasy. III. The language of patients with conversion hysteria, anxiety state and obsessive-compulsive neurosis. *J. Psychol.* 10:75, 1940.
3. Beck, S. J.: *Rorschach's Test, I: Basic Processes.* New York, Grune & Stratton, 1944.
4. Beck, S. J.: *Rorschach's Test, III: Advances in Interpretation.* New York, Grune & Stratton, 1952.
5. Bender, L.: *A Visual Motor Gestalt Test and Its Clinical Use.* New York, Research Monograph of the American Orthopsychiatric Association No. 3, 1938.
6. Computers in Psychiatry. *Psychiat. Ann.* 2, No. 12, December, 1972.
7. Cronbach, L. J.: *Essentials of Psychological Testing.* New York, Harper & Row, 1960.
8. Gesell, A.: *Gesell Development Schedules.* New York, Psychological Corporation, 1949.
9. Goldstein, K. and Scheerer, M.: *The Goldstein-Scheerer Test of Abstract and Concrete Thinking—The Object Sort.* New York, Psychological Corporation, 1951.
10. Good, P. and Brantner, J. P.: *The Physician's Guide to the MMPI.* Minneapolis, University of Minnesota Press, 1961.
11. Hathaway, S. R. and McKinley, J. C.: *Manual for Use of the Minnesota Multiphasic Personality Inventory.* New York, Psychological Corporation, 1951.

12. Harrower, M.: *Appraising Personality: An Introduction to the Projective Techniques.* New York, Clarion-Simon and Schuster, 1968.
13. Kent, G. and Rosanoff, A. J.: A study of word association in insanity. *Am. J. Insanity* 67: 37, 1910.
14. Klopfer, B. and Davidson, H. H.: *The Rorschach Technique: An Introductory Manual.* New York, Harcourt, Brace and World, 1962.
15. *Kuder Preference Record, Vocational Form G.* Chicago, Science Research Associates, 1956.
16. *Kuder Preference Record, Occupational Form D.* Chicago, Science Research Associates, 1956.
17a. Masserman, J. and Balken, Eva: The psychiatric and psychoanalytic significance of fantasy. Psychoanalyt. Rev. 26:343, 1949.
17. *Minnesota Paper Form Board Test.* New York, Psychological Corporation, 1970.
18. *Minnesota Clerical Test.* New York, Psychological Corporation, 1959.
19. Morgan, C. D., and Murray, H. A.: A method for investigating phantasies: The thematic apperception test. *Arch. Neurol. Psychiat.* 34:289, 1935.
20. Murray, H.: *Thematic Apperception Test Manual.* Cambridge, Harvard University Press, 1935.
21. Rorschach, H.: *Psychodiagnostics.* Trans. Lemkau, P. and Kronenberg, B. New York: Grune & Stratton, 1942.
22. Kotter, J. B.: *The Sentence Completion Test.* New York, Psychological Corporation, 1950.
23. Sargent, H. D. and Mayman, M.: Clinical psychology. *In* Arieti, S. (Ed.): *American Handbook of Psychiatry Vol. III.* New York, Basic Books, 1959.
24. Schwab, J. J.: *Handbook of Psychiatric Consultation.* New York, Appleton-Century-Crofts, 1968.
25. Strong, E. K.: *Strong Vocational Interest Test.* Palo Alto, Calif., Consulting Psychologists Press, 1959.
26. Wechsler, D.: *Wechsler Intelligence Scale for Children Manual.* New York, Psychological Corporation, 1949.
27. Wechsler, D.: *Wechsler Adult Intelligence Scale Manual.* New York, Psychological Corporation, 1955.
28. Wortis, S. B. and Halpern, F.: Psychological tests and indications for their use. *Med. Clin. N. Am.* 74: May, 1958.

Students who wish to obtain a more complete understanding of testing should refer to Cronbach's *Essentials of Psychological Testing*[7]; all students are urged to read Harrower's excellent book, *Appraising Personality: An Introduction to the Projective Techniques,*[12] which presents a lucid, exciting description of the clinical applicability of tests.

Chapter 7

EXAMINATION OF THE NONCOOPERATIVE PATIENT

Frequently, the psychiatric interviewer finds it necessary to examine non-cooperative, violent, negativistic or stuporous patients. Although the patient's inability to cooperate poses major obstacles, the examination provides an opportunity to assess alterations in his reactions as the clinical picture changes.

The basic considerations in the examination are: (1) observation, (2) the patient's reaction to stimuli, (3) the physical findings, and (4) special examinations. First, the interviewer should obtain the salient history of the present illness from relatives, other informants, or even police officers who may have brought the patient to the emergency room. The history-taking procedure, in such cases, should follow the outlines which have been described and should attempt to provide as complete an account as possible about the events which led to the present episode, the history of the present illness, personality characteristics, childhood development and familial background, a social history, and, importantly, questions concerning drug intake, alcohol, possible head injuries, and physical illnesses of various types.

LEVEL OF CONSCIOUSNESS

One of the interviewer's initial tasks when he is confronted with a noncooperative patient is to determine the level of consciousness. This exists on a continuum ranging from silent, vigilant or almost hyper-vigilant alertness through confusions or deliriums which are characterized by varying degrees of disorientation, clouding of consciousness characterized by a disturbance of attention and perception, stupor, or to coma—a state of near total or total unresponsiveness to the environment and to stimuli. The examiner can determine the level by observing the patient's facial expression, gait, posture, bodily activity, and his reactions to the stimuli of the physical examination. Catatonic patients, for example, may maintain a fixed, tight facial expression and a tension of the facial musculature even though their limbs can be moved into fixed positions (waxy flexibility or *cerea flexibili-*

tas). Hysteric patients may lie quietly on the examining table and may appear to be nonresponsive, but may resist the examiner's attempts to open their eyelids. Patients who have ingested various admixtures of drugs may lie quietly for a few moments and then burst spontaneously into a generalized outbreak of physical activity. Those who are in a post-ictal state may have had loss of sphincter control. In examining all noncooperative patients, the examiner should search for possible signs of cerebral trauma, evaluate the size and equality of the pupils and check their responses to light, and observe the patient's nasal and oral regions for evidence of alcohol or drugs. Tightly constricted pupils may be indicators of heroin overdosage, while in the more active patient, the presence of widely dilated pupils may signify a withdrawal reaction.

In essence, the observation of the patient should be focused on his facial expression, gait, posture, rigidity or flaccidity of the musculature, signs of possible brain injury or drug ingestion, excessive perspiration which may be indicative of anxiety or of a metabolic disturbance, dehydration and dryness of the tissues which may be found not only in patients with metabolic disturbances, but in addicts who are malnourished, presence or loss of sphincter control and, importantly, the state of the patient's clothing: is he neatly attired, carelessly dressed, or is there evidence of self-injury or trauma inflicted by others?

The violent patient's reactions should be carefully observed: Is he attempting to escape? Is he directing his violence toward a certain individual? Is he fragrantly aggressive? Or, is he just terribly frightened? In observing the violent or overactive patient's movements, the examiner can detect whether there is freedom of movement, the presence of injury to a limb or to the limbs on one side of the body, coordination, and other significant findings from the quality and quantity of motoric activity.

RESPONSE TO STIMULI

The examiner should undertake a systematic evaluation of the patient's responses to movement of the head, neck and limbs, to attempts to open or close the eyelids, and to the various procedures involved in the general physical and neurological examination.

Patients in hysterical or conversion or dissociated states, or those under the influence of drugs, or negativistic, mute, or catatonic schizophrenic patients may fail to respond to the "pin prick" or may suddenly overrespond. Attempting to gauge the patient's level of consciousness or to diagnose his condition solely from his response to painful stimuli, therefore, may be misleading; even delirious patients may respond erratically to such stimuli while withdrawn patients may regard such approaches as sadistic and become even more negativistic than previously.

The examiner may ask the mute patient to respond to questions by nodding, by lifting his hand, or by blinking his eyes. He may direct or command the patient to show his tongue, raise his limbs, walk about, or imitate movements, since this imitation (echopraxia) may be indicative of a brain lesion or of a schizophrenic state. He should offer the patient pencil and paper on which to write anything he wishes, particularly responses to questions which the examiner asks verbally, in writing, or in mime. The examiner should be acutely aware of the patient's general reactions to the environment and to certain individuals in the room. On occasion, a seemingly mute, noncooperative, resistent patient will begin to answer the examiner when relatives, the police, or others are removed from the room.

GENERAL PHYSICAL EXAMINATION

All noncooperative patients should be given a thorough physical examination. This involves careful inspection and palpation of the entire body, especially the head; a thorough examination of the eyes, ears, nose, and throat, including the fundi and the pharynx; inspection, palpation, percussion, and auscultation of the chest; examination of the abdomen for signs of abdominal rigidity and for either hypomotility or hypomotility of the intestines; examination of the limbs; rectal and pelvic examinations; and, in all instances, a complete neurological examination with tests for intactness of all the cranial nerves, sensation, and the reflexes. The examination should of course include temperature, pulse, and respiration, as well as blood pressure measurements from various extremities.

SPECIAL EXAMINATIONS

These include a urine analysis for possible evidence of diabetes, kidney disease, and especially the presence of drugs. A sample of blood should be drawn to determine the alcohol level as well as the routine blood chemistries and serologic examinations. When there is evidence of cerebral trauma, skull X-rays should be ordered as an emergency measure and, in many instances, a routine lumbar puncture should be performed, providing that there is no evidence of increased intracranial pressure as revealed by choked discs. On occasion, the contents of the patient's stomach should be obtained by gastric lavage for examination for drugs and poisons.

In summary, the examination of the noncooperative or inaccessible patient should be focused on observation, response to stimulation, general physical findings and the results of special examinations. In every instance, the patient should be examined by the doctor with a nurse or attendant in the room. Furthermore, the patient's behavior toward the examiner and toward other persons as well as the general environment should be carefully observed. Apparently meaningless behavior or various degrees of nonresponsivity during the examination of the acutely disturbed or seriously ill mental patient can reveal a great deal of information about his mental illness as well as the necessity of emergency treatment.

REFERENCES

1. Freedman, A. M. and Kaplan, H. I.: *Comprehensive Textbook of Psychiatry, Chapters 11–33*. Baltimore, Williams & Wilkins, 1967.
2. Kirby, George H.: *Guides for History Taking and Clinical Examination of Psychiatric Cases*. Albany, N.Y., The New York State Hospital Commission, 1921.
3. Mayer-Gross, W., Slater, E. and Roth, M.: *Clinical Psychiatry*. Baltimore, Williams & Wilkins, 1955 (pp. 43–52).
4. Miron, N. B. and Kalogerakis, M. G.: Chapters 24 and 25 *in* Masserman, J. H. (Ed.): *Current Psychiatric Therapies*, Vol. XIII. New York, Grune & Stratton, 1973.
5. Stevenson, I. and Sheppe, W. M.: The psychiatric examination. *In* Arieti, S. (Ed.): *American Handbook of Psychiatry*. New York, Basic Books, 1959 (pp. 213–234).

Chapter 8

THE PSYCHIATRIC EXAMINATION OF A CHILD

By Paul L. Adams, M.D.

Always unwilling to be cast into the role of psychiatric patients, children are frequently uncooperative. In Meyerian terminology, they are sometimes *resistive*—refusing to do what is asked of them—and sometimes *oppositional*—not only refusing to do what is asked but doing the diametric opposite. A child provides us with a highly instructive case of the unwilling patient. Children are not free to refuse the psychiatric evaluation, however, for children have a very weak legal status. They are technically owned by their parents until they have been legally emancipated from that bondage and set free, now, for most purposes, at 18 years of age. For legal reasons, if for no others, then, the child who is brought to the psychiatrist may be reluctant to cooperate, to talk, and to trust the strange grownup.

In this chapter we shall try to formulate some of the basic principles for beginning the psychiatric examination of children. These principles have to do with building a professional relationship with the child whose life problems and whose person are being studied. We shall cover in only a few pages (books already exist) the single hour of the first interview (thousands of lifetimes devoted to learning to help children have preceded us into the task) and attempt to order the topic into six subheadings—1) age appropriate outreach and play, 2) work with the child's parents, 3) testing and touching, 4) limitations of time and space, 5) goals of the first interview, and 6) strategies that facilitate the realization of the goals.

OUTREACH APPROPRIATE FOR THE CHILD'S SITUATION

The examining doctor will have to win the child's trust. The child has no background in carrying on a psychiatric interview. He knows only that this is a doctor to whom the child's parents insist that the child must go. He makes associations with pediatric care, and that means that even from a most benign pediatrician the prior care given the child often was frightening and painful. Hence, the unknown new doctor will seem even more threatening to the child, until the benign nature of the doctor has been demonstrated to the child. The child has no precognition that the psychiatric examination is not to be physically and mentally painful to him. The child needs to be shown the good "vibrations" of the benign and helping physician, lest he persist in his feeling alienated from and mistrustful of the doctor. A skilled interviewer can complete an accurate psychiatric evaluation of a child within a relatively short period of time.

Early on, the examiner should try to inform the child of his wish to help, of his identity as a medical student or doctor, and, if he is a psychiatrist, of his identity as a psychiatrist. It is important to ask the child what he would expect from a psychiatrist, what he has been told about the psychiatric interview, what has happened to him with other doctors, and to give some words of reassurance in conjunction with each question addressed to the child—that there will be no "shots" administered, that the session will be no longer than an hour's length, that the parents are either waiting nearby or are talking with a professional person in an adjacent room, or will be back to pick up their child at a specified time. Incidentally, it is always a good precaution to have at least one of the parents waiting for the child during the initial interview. Children often experience a relative abandonment and will be more readily congenial with a psychiatric interviewer whenever the interviewer can reassure the child of the easy proximity of the parents. Reassurance, verbal fluency and willingness to talk are paramount virtues within the first few moments of an initial interview with a child. Perhaps the cardinal rule in interviewing children is that *the interviewer must be active and verbal.* Children are turned off by those who try to be nondirective, aloof and "deep." Children see them as stingy withholders who are either scared or trying to unnerve the child. Silence between strangers can be an icy, hostile, and alienating phenomenon. Children do not fail to perceive that.

Grownups who do best in relating to children are grownups who have not brought down a total renunciation and repression of their own childhood experiences. That is, that person builds the best relationship who as an adult has not shunned childhood's Pure Delight (William Blake), the polymorphous hedonic revelry in all body parts (Norman O. Brown), or the Pleasure Principle (Sigmund Freud). Grownups who know the joys of play relate most easily to children as do grownups who have not stayed totally enculturated in the values of their parents, but who have moved aside enough in their participation that they could be said, in the Zen metaphor, to have "seen through" the conventions of their family and subculture. Grownups who relate best to grownups (radically and really) are the very ones who usually relate best to children. Mental health skills

required to carry on psychiatric work with children, and those who disclaim their helping competency with children are usually the selfsame people who lack that competency with adolescents, middle aged, and elderly
persons. Humanity in all its epochs and phases is no stranger to a good
doctor.

A generic empathy and brightness are needed for any and all psychiatric work. For work with children, more than with persons in any other age
group, there is an absolute necessity to operate with a *developmental
theory*. A developmental perspective makes the work lighter and more
fruitful. Children's problems and symptoms are sometimes devoid of their
richer meaning if they are not viewed within a developmental framework.
Even behavior modification practice utilizes a modicum of theory about
human development, seeing the human project in its entirety as one of
accommodation of each organism to an apparatus of pain-pleasure, or
reward-punishment. Family group therapy, while seldom child-focused,
operates with a rudimentary and general developmental theory, namely,
the view of Otto Rank that out of a primal symbiosis ("undifferentiated
ego mass"), the family's members are hatched and differentiated. Each
member of a family moves from absorption in collective experience to a
more specialized and individuated existence, the theory holds. Adlerian
theory stresses not only the birth of the Self but also of social feeling.
There are other theories that can be illuminating of the process of working
with and helping children. Perhaps one of the most useful is the largely
ethical neo-Freudian approach to the life cycle that has been explicated by
Erik Erikson,[1] or a related framework spelled out by Harry Stack Sullivan.[2]. The Developmental Profile of Anna Freud[3] is psychoanalytically
erudite. In a more exclusively cognitive mode is the developmental theoretical corpus advanced by Jean Piaget.[4] One can learn all of these and then
proceed as an eclectic, or one may join a school and remain faithful,
untroubled by the winds of change. But skeptical or faithful, *one must think
developmentally* if one is to do good work with children.

The preverbal two-year-old is in an existential setting that differs
starkly from the six-year-old who has become suddenly mute in response to
interpersonal stresses. And both of these are very different from the child
aged four years who has become steadily autistic and nonverbal. The
expert with children must be attuned to what the human stuff is all about,
and what characteristics are shared (some universally, some culture-wide,
and some only within subgroups bearing subcultures) by boys and girls of
specified sex and age. This assuredly, requires a knowledge of physical
growth norms but also of attitudinal and culturally variable norms. Against
a background mental image of the range of normality and deviance, the
adult interviewer busies himself to observe and evaluate the behavior of the

particular child whose fate he is sharing for a time. Knowing the expected norms and ranges only enhances the adult interviewer's discernment of all that is unique, personal and intrapsychic for the single child.

The two cardinal principles set down thus far are: the interviewer has to be outgoing and verbal. He reaches out to the child and wants to build a trusting relationship, but all the while he has a keen awareness of the child's developmental situation and the hurdles which stand in the way of the child's further progression.

Reaching out to children is done by the interviewer's active talking, active reassurance, and active offer of play. The interviewer also gets across, in an appropriate phrasing considering the child's age, that his singleminded purpose is to know the child's way of living, seeing, thinking, feeling and acting in the world. The interviewer can then question and test and take a history from the child as long as the child sees that the sole purpose is for the adult to see things from the child's viewpoint. Talk of school is often an easy conversation topic with children. School and play are their work, their vocation, and the way a child interacts and relates at school is appropriate for the adult to learn by visiting and direct observation. Children behave differently in groups of their agemates than they do with the most benevolent "shrinks," so school and other group settings should be observed if possible.

The watchword then, is to reach out and offer a willingness to see through the child's eyes, to stand in the child's shoes. That commitment in itself may be so novel that it will be astoundingly therapeutic in the initial session with a child. Not many adults, including many parents, communicate their zeal for empathy with a child. Hence, this empathic psychiatric style can introduce a really novel element into the child's world view.

In the context of our empathy for the child it becomes very sensible for us to want to ask him to report dreams (recent, recurrent and scariest), since we say that dreams represent a very personal, private form of thinking and doing. Likewise, the child cooperates when we ask him to draw things that he talks about; or to tell us what he likes and hates about various people in his intimate daily world; or to speak out his "associations" to certain conflicted topics; or to articulate his heart's three deepest wishes; or to share with us his very earliest memory, something he recalls (but not some scene he has been told about) that goes as far back as he can remember; or as we elicit his favorite teacher (along with the reasoning behind his favoring), his favorite friend, favorite animal, favorite joke, favorite famous person, etc.; or as we say, "Let's play a game where I will start saying sentences and you finish each one with the very first idea that pops into your head. What you say doesn't have to make sense. The main thing is to say it at once, as soon as I have started it." Empathy is a blood brother of enquiry, sharing and clarity.

WORKING WITH PARENTS AND CHILDREN

Usually the adults whom the child knows best are the adults whose attitudes he has incorporated in forming his own self-image, that is, the most important adults, his parents. Parents can be very constructive forces in a child's life. When a child is disturbed and having problems, however, the parents will often need help, shoring up, guidance, counseling, casework and sometimes even therapy. It is folly to try to figure out whether the parents or the child are to blame, because in psychiatric work we need not place blame. That is the job of a legal expert working in an adversary proceeding. We only help, listen, explore, and oftentimes undertake to free the parents as well as the child of the tyranny of *ought* and *should* under which they have grown up and under which they are bringing up their own children. Camilla Anderson,[5] a child psychiatrist, wrote most openly about moralistic hangups of parents and makes good reading for any grownup, with her advocacy of purging all morality from the people with whom we work before a true ethical sense can be developed. It is a matter, as William Penn wrote, of making ethical standards *our own*, instead of those of another person—a very fundamental task for anyone caring for children.

Parents are not patients. They come in with reality problems, centered in their child's troubles, and they have already made big growth strides by the time they have applied to us for help. There is little to be found blameworthy in such a step, so parents seeking help warrant our giving them respect and consideration.

Not only do parents own their child legalistically but also in a more "spiritual" sense they own their children: they see themselves in their children and they have confidence that the child is basically good—their "own." The psychiatric interviewer need not aspire to replace the real and lusty human relationships that flow between child and parents, for parents have the edge in all ways over the professional person who is interviewing and trying to help the child. Parents are real persons in the life and imagery of the child, whereas the doctor has a largely professional relationship with the child. The parental relationship, without being always engulfing and stifling, has a heartiness about it that no professional relationship can match. The child lives now with his parents, if the parents are alive and with him, and the parents to whom he relates are not merely "fantasy objects." They live and breathe, they love and hate, they tie up their children and each other in passionate bondings that make pallid, in comparison, the ties between a child and a professional healer. It is small wonder that the relation between a therapist and patient has been dubbed an "as if" relationship, not a "real objects" relationship.[6] The therapist can behave *as if* he were a parental figure to the child; but the parent *is* a parent, a begetter, a *source* out of which children do emerge and hatch, and come ultimately into an individuated existence with their own personalities.

Parents can be very helpful to our examination of the child. For example, they can prepare the child for the interview. What they say and how they say it can make or break the very first interview with the psychiatrist.

The very first contact with a child, as a result of this, often reveals (because it is sought after) the nature of the referral, what the parents told the child about the present appointment with the doctor, what kind of doctor the child expected to see, what other doctors the child has seen, what the other doctors are like and what the child felt about other doctors, and the difference between others and the present interviewer. Also the child is always asked about his "main problems" (or troubles; or things that bother him, upset him, make him unhappy; or that keep him from growing; or symptoms). Nothing supplants the child's own words about why he is there with us, and nothing can substitute for the child's own description of his developmental history nor his own view as to how he got to have the problems for which his parents (if not he or she) are seeking some help. The child seldom knows what "complaints" are as applied to his own life problems, so that word can safely be avoided. However, the best way to communicate is *to offer several terms* all at once, so the child sees that you are not trying for precision of speech but are only interested in trying for dialogue, self revelation and true interaction within the safeguards of a confidential, helpful, professional relationship.

Confidentiality is a specialized issue in work with children. Some excellent child psychiatrists do not bother themselves about confidentiality, buying into the idea that children are dependent beings whose parents had better be informed of anything and everything the doctor knows about their child. Others (including myself) hold to a dual standard, claiming that the child, being weaker and dependent, must know anything and everything that the parents say to the doctor but that the doctor will not betray any confidences between the doctor and the child. Sometimes I tell a child, "I will not squeal on you *unless* I have given you advance warning, so that you have a chance to talk me out of telling something to your parents. The only thing I would ever tell them, anyway, is something I am afraid you would do that would be harmful." When some children ask me for an example, I say "things like running off or breaking the law or doing something that would obviously only hurt you." The two extremes are no promises of confidentiality and a promise of total confidentiality, but there are other child psychiatrists who fall intermediately, sometimes divulging information and then trying to deal with the breaches in trust that are implicit in that. It should be added, however, that anyone consulting us who has made decisive steps toward emancipation from parents (adolescents, notably) deserves the same kind of strict confidentiality that an adult does. Most people who work with adolescents subscribe to this viewpoint, it seems, and never say anything to the parents behind an adolescent's back. This among other things has made family group therapy sessions particularly relevant to professional work with adolescents.

With preschool and elementary school children, more occasion for play is appropriate. What furnishings are needed for the child's play? As Melanie Klein[7] proposed, the consulting room "does not contain anything except what is needed for the psycho-analysis." I would suggest only a soft rubber ball, a gun, a doll family, and a pencil and paper. These, on a low table with two low chairs (one for interviewer and one for child), fill out the required furnishings. Anything else is *lagniappe*. Children have little interest in our credentials, diplomas, and the like; but their parents may if they are conscientious and well informed people.

The best way to do psychiatric interviewing with a child is to have seen the parents separately on an earlier occasion, and to see only the child in his session. After the first time they are seen by you the parents can be seen by your colleagues in medicine or social work or psychology. Alternatively, they may be interviewed in occasional family group sessions by you, but only when the child is present. Opinions vary about this issue.

When parents are seen without the child (and in advance of the child's being interviewed), some worthwhile psychiatric data can be uncovered. The following seem most useful: how they feel about coming to see you without their child, what they see as the child's major problems, how long the problems have existed, who other than the child seems most caught up in the suffering, why the parents sought help at this particular moment in time, what aggravates or lessens the problem, what the respective parents feel about the child, etc. I also like to ask them how their marriage and family first came about, and what major adjustments and reorientations or shifts have been made throughout the existence of the marriage. If the parents do not indicate that parenthood itself presented new challenges and crises, I ask them about their parenting, "What has fatherhood (or motherhood) meant to you as a person, married to this spouse?"

Some assessing and probing for parental intelligence, life style, "psychology-mindedness," motivation, empathy for their child, acceptance of anger and sexual lust, their intuitions about the final outcome of the child's difficulties—through all of these the parents are introduced to the work we do, and they provide us the information we need for doing our best work. We need a cooperative relationship with the child's parents; for they give us indispensable information, they help prepare the child for our evaluation and treatment, and they can facilitate (if everything goes well) the child's treatment in a sometimes-prolonged, secret and close relationship with a professional person. The parents have to get in shape to give more autonomy and freedom to their child. Slowly the realization comes to them that *what they are there for as parents* is to be sources of new, autonomous personalities. In return we can make the parents' lives as comfortable as possible, not always seeing them as patients but as parents, and also as man and wife, and also as autonomous, somewhat undomesticated persons themselves. Every child and his family are different, and can only be met and studied to be known. Our prejudices and counter-transferences do not work and will not help. Not all families are middle class like ours, or from our same religious background or with our same made-in-heaven origins and life style.

TESTING AND TOUCHING

Children come to live in a world of symbols very early, in culturogenic symbols and values. Language is not really developed well until the child reaches age three or more, and mushrooms only by age five or six years when the child is ready to go to school in a serious fashion. Children serve adult interviewers as happy reminders that we are contact-hungry animals, and that much of our gut-level communication occurs on a nonverbal basis. Gut level is not for the language of science, naturally, but scientific discourse is an elegant and acrobatic grace that comes with maturity alone. Children live in a world of close-up contacts. They smell, lick and taste, and they touch and stroke. They unabashedly like to be touched and petted, as a rule. Surely only an inhibited adult, with a crying need for derepression, would falter in making physical, bodily contact with a child patient. Sometime, however, it is only a light touch or gentle hug that a child is able to tolerate. It is best to proceed slowly, by stages, in touching disturbed children for after all they are somewhat unlike children who are not patients.

A doctor who has cuddled and comforted little children, and who is comfortable in touching children may be capable of a flexible stance concerning the physical examination of the child who is being evaluated in a *psychiatric* study. Many feel awkward in doing physical examinations, but others[8,9] have built opposing arguments that a physical exam can be an integrated and supremely elucidative portion of the child's psychiatric interview. If there is any rule at all to be discerned after witnessing the bitter feuding on the subject, it is probably to do what seems most helpful, professional and natural. If the patient will be convenienced or better helped by our performing a physical exam, it seems to be wise to do so.

Patient welfare should be put first, ahead of our dogmas and articles of faith. Furthermore, in a learning situation a good rule is to work as fully as possible within the limits and controls of the supervisory relationship. This kind of cooperation with the "system" has merit for the learning process; but it should never be carried too far. (*Too far* can be defined as blind acceptance, unquestioningly, of something taught a student in an authoritative way by an authoritarian teacher.) The student should cooperate in order to learn a given system but continue inquiring and learning.

Physical examination can be benign. Is the same thing true for psychologic testing, and other specialized measures to learn about the child?

Those of us who truly respect children, and who long to care for them, and who know that the first step toward professional helping is to see the world through the eyes of the child, will also feel easy about psychologic testing during the early sessions with a young person. Doctrinaire purists notwithstanding, the same person who wants to do psychotherapy can do diagnostic work too, including formal testing. No law, no logic, countermands psychologic testing. I prefer complete and accurate testing competently done by a qualified child psychologist. When that is a hard bill to fill, I do my own testing. The Vineland Social Maturity Scale, the vocabulary items from the Binet, the Bender Gestalt, the House-Tree-Person, the Kinetic Family Drawings, Squiggles, the appropriate cards from the Thematic or Children's Apperception Test—all are within the ken of the average rushed medical student or psychiatric resident. I personally use the Sentence Completion Game frequently and, as time goes by, the Rorschach only rarely. For the latter a "real psychologist" is better. When their results are judiciously weighed and balanced against all the other data derived from the early sessions with a child, they facilitate working with children, for they give useful baseline data for later comparisons, and they help in the diagnostic effort.

TIME AND SPACE LIMITS

Every interview with a child is a finite experience, a professional relationship, that is, a relationship that will end when enough helping or teaching or self-growth has taken place. The child knows the interviewer not as a parent or an uncle or aunt: the relationship limits the amount of cravings that will flow back and forth between adult and child. The relationship is impeded by "transference analysis" at every turn. The child knows and is often reminded that this is a relationship to be studied, talked about and compared to other relationships, such as those with his parents, siblings, teacher, priest, other doctors, and so on. Sometimes, for the first time a child can take some pleasure from a relationship that is not a bondage.

That it is a limited relationship can also be suggested in the very first hour, as the interviewer tells the child "We will go to my workshop (office/ consulting room/playroom) for about an hour where we will do some talking and drawing; then you will be back here with your mommy." The child sees that there are limits on his time with the doctor, and that these are definite, not easily pushed around. Or, to take another example, some child psychiatrists employ a routine course of telling their child patients that the first 25 minutes is for work, the last 25 for play and refreshment. This adopts some of the attentiveness to time and place that the school child lives with in his daily working world. As soon as it has happened, I also tell a child who comes late for an appointment that I simply cannot make up for time that he misses due to lateness, but that since I am responsible and accountable for what I do I *will* make up any of my own tardiness at times that are convenient for the child and the parents.

Still another way that we set the tone of a limited, professional relationship with a child is to charge the parents for the work we do. This aspect of medical money-making has often been stressed too much. There are countries other than the US where under socialized medicine such services are free for those who need them, with the professional person being paid through other mechanisms than the fee-for-service plan. Nonetheless, when the family is paying rather dearly for the hours the child spends with a psychiatrist, the psychiatrist can often see that some of the "waste not, want not" morality gives a boost to the limiting, limited, professional relationship between the child and the interviewer. Where money is charged for the sessions, the child and the parents must be involved in talk, originally and repeatedly, about the fee set; for only in that way can it come into the open as a reality issue.

Young children are closer to adults than to adolescents in one way— their use of time during the early interviews. Before they are adolescent, children open up and reveal some of their basic orientations and conflicts during the very first interview. The adolescent, however, is a little more complex. What the adolescent shows is not so often his entire self. Hence, I need to see adolescents for three or four sessions before I can feel that I have had a sufficient sampling of their roles, selves, possibilities. Three or four half-hour sessions are almost as fruitful in providing the needed panoramic sample as are three or four sessions of an hour's length. Oftentimes, a young woman will come across as a hoyden one time, a madonna another, again borderline psychotic, again a sufferer of "amotivational syndrome." The four have to be put on the scales, undergo a balanced assessment, and then be summarized in a way that will do full justice to the young woman. One of the most common snares for male medical students is to promote the seductive and histrionic "face" of an adolescent woman during the first session, only to be astounded at the next session by the "serious pathology" or sexless austerity of the same young woman who came on so "captivatingly" (flirtatiously) the first hour.

The adolescent male presents the same diagnostic challenge to an adult interviewer of either sex. The young man also oscillates and vacillates from one mask to another, and from mood to mood, requiring more than one or two visits to be seen or understood. A therapeutic relationship with an adolescent is assuredly not to be built in a day.

GOALS OF THE FIRST HOUR

In the first hour with a child some positive developments can occur. Indeed these positive developments are to be aimed for, and without being grandiose we should feel that something has been accomplished on each of the following counts[10]:

1. positive relatedness of child to adult
2. diagnostic formulation
3. preliminary appraisal of treatability
4. beginning of treatment planning

Relatedness is fostered when the adult begins by talking and giving to the child in the waiting room, and as he stoops down to the child's level and expresses a real interest in knowing what it is like to live in this world, seeing the world through the eyes of the child. By offering help, or stating his wish to know and help the child, the adult wins something in the direction of trust and confidence on the part of his young friend. As he explains and structures the session, giving the child not only a chance to talk but also encouraging the child to live up to his obligation to talk, the adult helps to move the relationship to one of positive rapport.

The child sees the adult as someone who (even a bit oddly) asks his opinions about everyday events, expresses interest in the child's family and how he sees his kinfolk, shows a lively concern in the schoolwork and play of the child, and acknowledges that the child has an important inner life of fantasy and perceptions. For some children this kind of respect has never been encountered before in any adult the child has known, and the child derives reassurance and comfort even from the adult's very investigative work of questioning and trying to understand. Once that ice has been broken, the adult interviewer can be forgiven some egregious blunders (if they are not made habitually), for the child knows the adult's heart and head are both in the right places.

A *diagnostic formulation* does not have to be a perfectly polished and honed product. By the end of the initial session it is often highly tentative, and may be so speculative and off-course that the note on the first interview looks a little strange after a few weeks of familiarity have elapsed. Still, one session is enough to get us started in our diagnostic task. Usually by the end of the first hour we can say whether the child we have spent the hour with is out of contact with us, whether he is deeply troubled, whether he has a rather fixed psychopathologic structure, whether he seems overwhelmed by situational stresses, whether he shows signs of central nervous disorder, whether he has a cognitive dysfunction such as mental retardation, whether he has a character problem, or is healthy, etc. Piecing together what the child has presented and blending that with what the parents or the referral agents have told us, we can begin to make a pretty plausible story for the child's predicament. We can not only assess the severity but also have some idea of the developmental significance of his problems, as well as competencies and successes. We know something of the onset, the precipitant stresses, the premorbid level of adjustment, and the areas of his developing self which have remained relatively strong and non-pathologic. We know who other than the child is bound up in the syndrome—the interpersonal significances and ramifications of being a disturbed (and disturbing) child in a small group, the family.

Some preliminary appraisal of the child's treatability can be hoped for after the first interview. Our knowledge, still being acquired, of the severity and fixity and variety of the child's difficulties is further enlarged by our knowledge of the parental situation, the assets and liabilities of the parent or parents. The onus, in adjudging treatability, is seldom on the child. For I am convinced[11] that other elements are equally determinative of treatability: the referral, the parents, the siblings, the community resources, the interviewer himself and the facility in which the helping professional operates. Often that spectrum of factors outweighs what the child has within him. Therefore, in order to evaluate the child's treatability we should consider more than simplistic concerns with money or middle classness, education, fluency in English, whiteness, and the family's zeal in adopting the ideology of depth psychotherapy. These are all reality circumstances, but children who do not have any of the money-related attributes just listed make exemplary candidates for psychiatric assistance, including psychotherapy.

The beginning of treatment planning should *not* be done before the first session with the child. All too often, people in the mental health field have a narrow repertoire of helping acts, and before they have even seen a child they have postulated that the child may not be treatable *by them*. Such therapists need some lessons in diversification and flexibility, in humanism and the commitment to meet human needs. Otherwise, they will go on through life articulating self-fulfilling prophecies about the untreatability of certain kinds of children. The children's worth is not so much in question as that of the evaluating professional.

The student learning the basic approaches and techniques should be willing to project the most optimistic and ideal treatment plans, knowing that they are optimal, and assuming for a while that we live in a society devoted to human services. So the first move in planning a treatment regimen should consider what would be ideally helpful if money, distance, etc., did not interfere. Only secondarily, should the student begin to think in practical terms, seeking manageable trimmings and modifications on the ideal plan to help the given child and family. In all of medicine, and in the more specialized but at the same time broader and interdisciplinary field of mental health, the bowing to practical but second-rate arrangements is like a reflex for us who live in the concrete world of practicality and empiricism.

A child who is suffering from an obsessional neurosis, for example, should have psychotherapy freely available to him, but in addition the family may need subsidy if they are poor, the child may need remedial tutoring for his academic hangups and deficiencies, and a more energetic sports or recreation program for his stilted bodily habitus and rigid muscular "armor." Further, he will almost certainly need good medical care either from a pediatrician or a family doctor, or from the child psychiatrist under some circumstances. Children do not know that they are supposed to present problems in pure culture, so they frequently come in for psychiatric evaluation with an admixture of health problems, educational problems, welfare problems, reality problems and fantasy problems. A skillful treatment plan does not overlook any areas of a child's needs.

SUMMARY OF INTERVIEW STRATEGIES

Children are dependent and emergent human beings. They consume security, and adults provide it, so aloofness or neutrality is ridiculous with a child. Children have inner lives, rich in fantasy, with room for play, and for ecstasy if they are not overly programmed and regimented. They have the facility to communicate both nonverbally and verbally. They dream, they have urges and impulses, and they have hangups that are socially patterned but sometimes quite idiosyncratic. To work with children we need an ideology containing a developmental perspective; we also need a sociocultural perspective that allows us to study and accept differences in life styles; and we need to have a zeal to understand the way the child lives "from inside outward."

Given that kind of a humanistic outlook, and some simple technology —defined as "know how"—we are ready to be skillful interviewers and helpers of children. The *materials* are very simple ones, toys and paper and pencil, and a contract-like arrangement that the child will be there at a certain time and place, perhaps on a recurrent and regular basis, and that the parents too will stay involved in the changes that their child will need to be making for his own betterment. In addition to basic supplies, the *space* of an office (or home, since home visits are excellent techniques) and some *know how and ideology*, we probably have to have good *supervision* in the early stages of our learning to work with children. Nothing can replace personal tutelage when we are learning to work with children, and as most psychiatrists know very well, even the finished product, a Psychiatrist, fares better if he keeps turning to his colleagues for counsel and sharing as he continues through life, open to incessant learning.

The strategies that work best with a child are strategies that are not overly complex, but simple and direct. Concrete examples are better than wordy and abstruse intellectualizings. Using many terms or words to make a point is superior to pontifical questions, or precise lawyer-like interrogation. Interpretations and clarifications that are given tentatively are better than assertions that bring about the child's airtight entrapments, for a child who is caught redhanded is more likely to be guilty and resentful than to achieve a healing insight. To be active and verbal, and giving, without being doctrinaire and intrusively disrespectful is what is required. By touching the child as he seems to want it, and by being eclectic and always attuned to supplying the child's wants and shortages within a professional relationship, we will be more natural and helpful than if we are the opposite kind of professional person. It is our aim to further the child's gratifications, not ours. Children welcome our calling a spade a spade and they quickly come to appreciate an unhinting directness, a getting right down to cases with a doctor whose benevolence has been proved to them.

REFERENCES

1. Erikson, Erik H.: Growth and crises of the health personality. *Psychological Issues* 1: 50-100, 1959.
2. Sullivan, Harry S.: *Conceptions of Modern Psychiatry*. New York, W. W. Norton, 1953.
3. Freud, Anna: *Normality and Pathology in Childhood: Assessment of Development*. New York, International Universities Press, 1965.
4. Piaget, Jean: *The Construction of Reality in the Child*. New York, Basic Books, 1954.
5. Anderson, Camilla: *Saints, Sinners and Psychiatry*. Portland, Ore., Durham Press, 1950.
6. Tarachow, Sidney: *An Introduction to Psychotherapy*. New York, International Universities Press, 1963.

7. Klein, Melanie: The psychoanalytic play technique. *In* Klein, M. et al. (Eds.): *New Directions in Psychoanalysis*. New York, Basic Books, 1955.
8. Levy, David M.: Method of integrating physical and psychiatric examination with special studies of body interest, overt protection, response to growth and sex differences. *Amer. J. Psychiat.* 9: 121, 1929.
9. Schonfeld, William: Body-image in adolescents: a psychiatric concept for the pediatrician. *Pediatrics* 31: 845, 1963.
10. Committee on Therapy, Group for the Advancement of Psychiatry: *Reports in Psychotherapy: Initial Interviews.* GAP Report Number 49. New York, GAP Publications Office, 1957.
11. Adams, Paul L.: *A Primer of Child Psychotherapy*. Boston, Little, Brown, 1973.

Additional

12. Gordon, R. A.: Understanding Children. New York, Science House, 1973.
13. Freedman, A. M. and Kaplan, H. I.: *The Child,* Vol. II. New York, Science House, 1973.

Chapter 9

REVIEW OF THE PRINCIPLES AND TECHNIQUES
OF THE PSYCHIATRIC EXAMINATION:
GUIDE TO FORMULATION

Rationale

Adverse life experiences, if severe and prolonged, may lead both to organic disorders and deviant social conduct. Therefore, no clinical evaluation is complete unless it includes (1) the patient's current psychologic and interpersonal as well as physiologic dysfunctions (present illness), (2) the nature and severity of the stresses that precipitated or exacerbated these decompensations (recent etiology), (3) the constitutional and experiential vectors that rendered the patient vulnerable to the specific stresses (remote etiology, personality traits), and (4) the prospects of his responding favorably or unfavorably not only to medical and surgical treatment, but also to spontaneous or directed interpersonal and environmental readaptations (prognosis and therapy). An interview is, eloquently, an interpersonal exchange of views leading to mutual insights.

The Psychiatric Attitude

The examiner will remember, from his own training and personal experiences, that under special life situations he himself had occasionally reacted with excessive anxieties, obsessive suspicions and fears, minor depressions, and other deviations in thinking and mood with their accompanying physiologic and behavioral expressions. Empathy so engendered will contribute to professional tact and understanding, sharpen the examiner's sensitivity to important clinical data, promote communication and confidence and thus, even in the first interview, lay the groundwork for effective therapy. Special interest and practice in the psychiatric aspects of a comprehensive diagnosis will eventually facilitate more rapid comprehension of essentials in the individual case, but until such skill is attained it is well to proceed in a thorough and orderly fashion in general accordance with this outline.

Objectives

With rapport established as above, the examiner can proceed to elicit the following data:

The present illness, comprising the patient's complaints, supplemented by a directed inquiry as to other significant symptoms and the circumstances which precipitate, exacerbate or relieve them.

The personality profile, as derived from a historical survey of the patient's *characteristic patterns* during his early childhood, in his schooling, and in his sexual, social, occupational, and other relationships. The nature of previous maladaptations to environmental stress and frustration or to bodily disease are to be noted, especially with regard to the events that precipitated and complicated the present illness.

The mental status, as deduced from his directly observed speech and behavior, and his responses to special tests.

Dynamic Formulation

Valid deductions from the anamnestic data as to (a) the patient's physical and intellectual endowment (b) his acquired character traits, including special capacities and vulnerabilities, and (c) the weight of other factors relevant to prognosis and therapy.

The clinical methods to be employed in securing this information must be varied to suit each patient, but the following procedure will be found generally applicable.

THE PRESENT ILLNESS

In many instances the patient, even after psychiatric referral, may still believe himself to be physically ill and initially resent any implications that his symptoms have other than a primarily organic causation. It is often advisable, therefore, to confirm the usual systemic history and physical and laboratory procedures not only as an essential preliminary and differential diagnostic step to enhance the patient's cooperation, but in the further investigation of pyschiatric factors. Conversely, since a diagnosis of neurosis or psychosis can never be made "by excluding organic disease," but must instead be based on psychiatrically positive data, it is well to look for such evidence fairly early in the diagnostic survey. Thus, with the medical findings reasonably complete, the patient may be tactfully but objectively informed that, happily, there is little or no indication of bodily disease, but that his symptoms could spring from other causes that also require thorough consideration. Relatively neutral and acceptable terms suitable to the individual case (e.g., "overwork," "prolonged worry," or "emotional strain," etc.) may be employed in these introductory explanations, but it is best to avoid confusing or accusatory phrases such as "psychosomatic disorder," "nervous breakdown," "neurosis," or "mental illness." Most patients, if they are thus made to feel that the examiner is understanding and sympathetic, will more readily accept the possibility of so-called "functional" or "emotional" elements in their illness, after which their examination may be continued as follows:

Review of the Presenting Complaints

Often these will be typical of significant psychiatric syndromes:

Anxiety states: characterized by recurrent episodes of precordial palpitation, shallow or catchy respiration, pounding pulse, sweating, tremulousness and intense subjective apprehension, with or without a feeling of a lump or obstruction in the throat (globus hystericus), urinary urgency, splanchnic constriction ("butterflies in the stomach"), giddiness or similar symptoms. Patients often complain of these as "heart attacks," "fainting spells," etc., but in most cases the symptoms are unrelated to exertion (as in cardiac decompensation), dietary factors (as in hypoglycemia), heat intolerance (as in hyperthyroidism) or other physical stress, and so obviously precipitated or relieved by emotional factors that the differential diagnosis need not be difficult.

Depressive syndromes: with insomnia, anorexia or occasional bulimia, variable constipation, easy fatigability, impotence in males and dysmenorrhea in women, and variable subjective complaints of inability to concentrate, discouragement, hopelessness, hypochondriacal preoccupations, fixed melancholy, or in severe cases, thoughts of and attempts at suicide. Intercurrent episodes of forced cheerfulness and distracting hyperactivity may or may not be truly hypomanic; in most instances, there is little true euphoria, and such reactions merely represent efforts to deny and overcompensate for the underlying anxiety and depression.

Phobic-obsessive-compulsive syndromes: comprising fears (phobias) partially recognized as irrational, unwelcome but insistent and recurrent (obsessive) thoughts or fantasies, and ritualized behavior patterns (compulsions) which, when prevented or frustrated, are replaced by feelings of intense anxiety.

Epileptic equivalents, even in the absence of grand or petit mal convulsions, may be suspected on the basis of episodes of clouded thinking, momentary bewilderments or confusions ("absences"), or transient fuguelike automatism, with or without post-dromal amnesia, fatigue and headache.

Toxic-delerious states due to drugs (including alcohol and narcotics) or intercurrent infections may be surmised from severe confusions, rapidly changing hallucinatory experiences, ataxias and other motor distrubances and distorted recall.

Psychotic admixtures are revealed by bizarre ideation, gross illogicality, extreme and protracted deviations in mood or seriously altered rapport, or pathognomic symtoms such as persistent hallucinations, grandiose and paranoid delusions and markedly impulsive behavior.

Impairments of cortical function, indicated by variable loss of memory (especially recent), perceptive integrations, inadaptability to new or unusual tasks, and progressive deterioration of personal and social habits.

Techniques of Inquiry

There are, of course, many other psychiatrically significant configurations; the above are presented only as a reminder of the fairly common syndromes that can be revealed by an exploration of the presenting semeiology. In this exploration, however, certain precautions should be followed, e.g.:

Specificity of description: Record the patient's complaint in his own terms, since his choice of language may be both evasive and illuminating. When, for instance, a patient complains of "headache" he may have no actual cephalalgia, but may instead mean a sense of inertia, or emptiness, or oppressive feelings, or other generalized discomforts vaguely referred to his "head." Other terms favored by patients because of their obscurity are "dizziness" (ranging from vertigo and slight faintness to syncope), "noises in the head" (tinnitus to obsessive sounds to auditory hallucinations), "nervousness" (meaning anything from mild restlessness and hypersensitivity to uncontrolled furors), "sleeplessness," "irritability," "tension," etc.

Tact: Some patients may have special guilts or sensitivities and cannot be pressed too intensely at their first interview without invoking anxiety and resentment. If such patients show obvious resistances, do not insist on an immediate inquisition into confidential or guarded material such as secret drinking, sexual deviations, parental attitudes, etc. Indications of the importance of these parameters may be evident, but their further explorations may be postponed until the patient's confidence has been more securely won.

Circumstances that exacerbate or alleviate the presenting complaints: Information as to symptomatology can in most cases easily be obtained merely by a receptive attitude or a few evocative questions; in fact, the number and variety as well as the nature of the complaints poured forth under such circumstances may in itself be indicative of a psychiatric admixture. When, however, it is necessary to make further inquiry as to the relationships of the patient's symptoms to inner emotional stresses, greater circumspection and skill are called for. Once secured, the following data may be highly significant:

Typical settings in which anxiety, phobias, obsessions, etc., are evoked: e.g., when the patient is called upon to perform an unwanted task, when he is reprimanded by some authority, or when he is otherwise rendered fearful, helpless or hostile.

Possible correlations for an otherwise unaccountable *periodicity* in the patient's symptomatology: a wife's migraine headaches which appear only on weekends when she must contend with the continuous presence of her husband and children, or recurrent impotence in a husband who unconsciously wishes to avoid impregnating his wife during her presumably fertile sexual cycle.

The *nature* of the symptoms may be revealing, e.g.: gastrointestinal dysfunctions in immature, dependent patients, under circumstances in which they feel suddenly frustrated and angry. However, in the absence of specific evidence, care must be taken not to make untenable presumptions about "specific psychosomatic formulas."

The circumstances under which symptoms are *relieved* may likewise be important: vacations, change of work or home, alterations in the family or social constellation, hospitalizations, and so on.

Particularly significant is the history that the patient had felt initially benefited by a *wide variety of treatments* administered by many doctors, but that in each case the "illness" returned as the physician's enthusiasm flagged, after which the patient would seek another with renewed complaints. This, of course, has a prognostic bearing on the patient's relationships and responses to therapy.

Preliminary information may likewise be gathered about the deliberate or covert advantages the patient may derive from his illness. These may take the form not only of financial compensation and relief from responsibilities ("secondary gain"), but may also satisfy security-seeking, regressive, covertly aggressive and other "primary" neurotic purposes.

Precipitation of the present illness: Whenever possible, the examiner should determine special circumstances which, operating on a previously sensitized individual, served to precipitate his current symptoms. In the case of combat or postcatastrophic neuroses the trauma may be fairly obvious, but more frequently, though the stresses involved were taken just as seriously by the patient, they are far less evident to an outside observer. In such instances they may consist of more subtle but equally disruptive threats such as a dreaded demotion or promotion, guilt over the secretly desired illness of a rival, an impending engagement or marriage, or various social or religious events or transgression of unique symbolic significance to the patient. Inquiry into such causes must be especially skillful, but is often highly illuminating.

THE PERSONAL HISTORY

Since psychiatric disorders are exacerbations of previously latent behavior tendencies, it follows that every neurotic or psychotic illness is an outgrowth of the patient's previous personality, and that the formation of the latter must be traced as fully as practicable from early familial influences through the vicissitudes of later life to the onset of his current disabilities. Training and practice in this task will make it far less formidable and time-consuming than it first appears, but here, as elsewhere in the psychiatric examination, the examiner must remember that many patients will be ignorant of, and unconsciously resist recognizing, any connection between their current difficulties and certain cherished attitudes and behavior patterns derived from their past experiences. This may be particularly true when crude or even merely routine attempts are made to elicit the familial and personal history; under such circumstances the patient may well defend himself, verbally or covertly, with some rationalization such as: "I came here for relief from headaches and bowel trouble, and they send me to a mental clinic where I'm asked if my grandmother was insane, and whether I really love my wife! Am I crazy?" Such reactions may be avoided only if the patient is given a preliminary understanding of the importance of a past history in arriving at a better diagnosis and more effective therapy, and if the interview continues to be conducted with proper empathy and adroitness. These considerations are helpful:

Interview Arrangements: Whenever practicable, choose a quiet, preferably soundproof office free of distractions and interruptions. The furnishings should be homelike rather than austere, and a few diplomas among the paintings on the walls help comfort the patient. Reassure him that all data will be kept professionally confidential.

Note-Taking: The examiner should be sufficiently familiar with the nature of the information he seeks to make it unnecessary to consult this or any other outline during the examination; to do so implies incompetence and impairs the ease, rapport and effectiveness of the relationship. For the same reasons, it is best to avoid voluminous writing (or covert audio recording) during the interview, but brief notes may be taken of key facts and expressions for later elaboration.

Transitions in Content: If the patient has, during his account of the present illness, vaguely or euphemistically described himself as "nervous," "emotional," "over-sensitive," "high-strung," etc., it may later be asked if these or other characteristics were familial traits, thus leading the patient to give significantly colored descriptions of his relationships with his parents, relatives and siblings under the guise of "the family history." Similarly, logical transitions may be made from the present illness to various categories of the past by inquiry as whether current or other symptoms were present in childhood, and whether they were influenced by "excessive study in school," "overwork," other maladjustments at early jobs, or the stresses of various social adaptations, and so on. Information on particularly guarded topics such as sexuality may be more readily secured by an indirect anamnestic approach: a complaint of dysmenorrhea may be used as a basis for asking the patient to describe the circumstances of her menarche; once the subject is broached, she may be more easily led to describe her initial fears and fantasies, sexual "traumata" and possibly neurotic reactions. Similarly, tracing a complaint of ejaculatio praecox in a male patient may reveal familial prohibitions of sex activity and later fears of masturbation or homosexuality directly related to his present marital or other difficulties.

"Irrelevancy." On the other hand, the patient's tendencies to surface diffuseness or seeming evasiveness when given an opportunity to talk spontaneously and freely—as should be done insofar as practicable—may in themselves be directly significant if basic associative themes are detected. For example, a patient may "wander" quite significantly from an account of her marital unhappiness to a description of her idyllic childhood with her widowed mother, or an aggressively competitive individual may "inadvertently" touch on his own multiple superiorities to others, including, by implication, the examiner. With limited time, a completely undirected interview is rarely as informative as a skillfully guided one, but both techniques may be used as indicated by the experienced examiner.

Sources of the Personal History: In general, the patient himself is the most fertile and significant source for the needed data, but wherever necessary or available, other sources may be used: interviews with family and friends, perusal of physicians', employers', or social service reports, school or military records, etc. It must be remembered, however, that all such sources have various limitations and biases so that each may require individual evaluation and check against the others.

Significance of the Data: It will be recognized that a psychiatric history is not merely a chronological account of the patient's life, but an attempt to discern those *characteristic patterns of behavior* which constitute his personality, and, therefore, possess psychiatric diagnostic and prognostic value. The aim, therefore, is not only to determine *what happened* in the patient's life, but also (a) his role in bringing the original occurrences about, (b) his subsequent responses to them, and (c) how, consciously or not, he arranged for the repetition of similar experiences. Thus, there need be no overt striving for a precise "historic accuracy" since if the patient's own accounts of past events are deliberately falsified, distorted, or even replaced by symbolic ("screen") memories, his *patterns* of communication will be psychiatrically significant. In this sense, the proffered "history" is in itself an excellent index of the patient's mental status, in that it furnishes valuable data as to his motivations, fantasies, self-concepts, and current interpersonal relationships.

With these techniques and qualifications, the information secured under the heading of personal history may be grouped under the following categories:

The Family History. It is highly questionable whether there are significant hereditary factors in neurotic or many psychotic disorders; however, it is undeniable that the personality of every adult is greatly influenced by those with whom he comes into intimate contact in childhood. Therefore, even apart from its genetic significance, the patient's own description of the personal characteristics of his grandparents, parents, siblings, or other relatives is often significant, particularly when special aspects of, or gross deviations in, their behavior (overindulgence, tyranny, unpredictability, neglect, tempestuousness, sexual seduction, etc.) directly affected the patient's early formative experiences. Note also his subsequent allegiances or aversions to parent-surrogates, such as governesses or teachers, attachments to and rivalries with various siblings, and the adverse influences of familial discord, divorce, or desertion.

Birth and Early Development: Accurate data may be difficult or impossible to obtain, but the patient's or other informants' impressions about the following may be significant: prematurity; ease or difficulty in delivery (asphyxia, injuries); type of nursing and methods of weaning; delays in early habit acquisitions such as sitting, walking, word or sentence formations, and toilet training; play interests; manifestations of early neurotic tendencies such as feeding difficulties, excessive crying, night terrors, tics, spasms, phobias, persistent thumb sucking or enuresis, etc.

Schooling and Initial Socialization: Ages of enrollment and at various grades attained; adjustment to school routine and discipline; scholastic and extracurricular activities liked and disliked; development, nature and depth of leadership or group loyalties at various ages; and unusual dependence upon or friction with teachers or other school authorities. School phobias, repeated disciplinary difficulties, social isolations, truancies and delinquencies are especially significant (as supplemented by play, games, or other techniques). The above data are, of course, particularly relevant in the direct or ancillary examination of children and early adolescents.

Sexual Development and Attitudes: Tactful, objective inquiry into early sex preoccupations (autoerotisms, curiosities, fantasies, fears, inhibitions, displacements); later development; nature pace and intensity of homo- or heterosexual expressions; deviations in technique or unusual attachments or aversions to sex partners. Previous and current marital adjustments including not only sexual compatibility, but also relative fidelity or promiscuity, use and justification of contraceptive methods, attitudes to in-laws and children, mutual interests and other interpersonal conflicts and satisfactions. In most cases, it will be found that these considerations *secondarily* determine sexual adjustments in marriage, rather than vice versa.

Other Habit Developments: concerning food, sleep, dress, hobbies, recreations, etc. In later life, the survey should include habitual overindulgence in tobacco, caffeine drinks, alcohol and, in recent years, "tranquillizers," barbiturates ("downers"), stimulants ("uppers"), "psychedelic" drugs ("pot," LSD, mescaline, hashish) or even addictive narcotics.

General Social Adjustments: Type and constancies of friendships and group loyalties and submissiveness or leadership in joint activities. Nature and intensity of significant social, ethical and religious sentiments, with special reference to unusual rigidities or prejudices. Circumstances leading to compatibility and belongingness, or, conversely, feelings of shyness, diffidence, embarrassment, resentment, alienation, and social failure.

Occupational History: Types of work sought or idealized; jobs secured and periods held; variability of effort and application; acceptance of duties and cooperation, or competitiveness with fellow workers; idleness and failures, responses to supposed injustice, or to promotions and successes; evaluation of employers, superiors or employees.

Military Service: Dates; branch; reactions to training, discipline and combat; demotions and promotions; type, grade and motivations at discharge; pensions sought and retained; current attitudes.

Social History: Basic information about the patient's socioeconomic background, including father's and mother's occupations, educational attainments, and aspirations for their children. The examiner should also elicit information about particular cultural or subcultural attitudes toward life in general, illness, and medical care. From this part of the anamnesis the examiner can determine the patient's social mobility (the strain which may accompany achievement and upward mobility or the sense of failure accompanying downward social mobility), sentiments, values, prejudices, and particular subcultural attitudes.

Effects of Injuries and Illness: An account of the patient's previous organic illnesses, including a description of significant reactions to them such as excessive invalidism, prolonged disability and dependency or lack of cooperation with medical care. Accident-proneness and consequent litigation may also be significant. Note all hospitalizations.

Transition to Present Illness: Under this heading the pyschiatric anamnesis may be completed by a consideration of the circumstances that, singly or in combination as outlined above, interacted with the patient's special sensitivities and vulnerabilities to precipitate his present illness, and later, to seek (or be referred for) psychiatric help. Not infrequently, however, a complete demarcation cannot really be made, and the "present illness" will be seen as merely a continuation, or, at most, an exacerbation of the patient's previous life patterns and aberrant tendencies.

THE CURRENT ("MENTAL") STATUS

Direct Observation: In most previous guides for psychiatric history-taking, a great deal of emphasis was placed on this portion of the psychiatric examination, since it was intended to reveal gross deviations in motivation, affect, thinking, and behavior relevant to the differential diagnosis of various forms of "mental deficiency," "pyschopathy," or organic and "major" psychoses. The examiner must, of course, remain alert to these possibilities; however, a far larger number of his subjects will have only characterologic, neurotic, or functional somatic disturbances, and in these, direct and crude investigations of intellectual capacities, disorientations, or hallucinatory experiences may be not only unnecessary but needlessly disturbing and alienating. Actually, valid information as to most of the rubrics of the so-called "mental status" will already have been gathered during the course of the history and physical examination, as will be indicated by the following review.

General Behavior: As manifested by the patient's appearance, gait, posture, demeanor, dress, personal hygiene, mannerisms, tics, characteristic activity, manifest idiosyncracies or compulsions, cooperation with office or clinic procedures, and general responses to the examiner and others.

Intellectual Level: This may be deduced fairly well from the quickness and relevance of the patient's preceptions, the versatility and specificity of his vocabulary, his capacities for both concrete and abstract thinking, the scope and accuracy of his general information, the richness of his imagery, his forms of wit and humor, and the general nature of his cultural attainments. In estimating basic intellectual capacities, however, allowances must be made for the previous presence or absence of social and educational opportunities.

Sensorium: Memory, retention, associative and communicative capacities, orientation, etc., are not organically impaired in the neuroses. If, however, intellectual failures possibly due to cerebral trauma, disease or dysrhythmia, are indicated by gross discrepancies in dates, places and relationships in the history, the patient's sensorium may be further checked by indirect questions designed (ostensibly as a test of "concentration," "alertness," etc.) to reveal his awareness of identity, time and locale, his capacity to remember his past consistently, to repeat forward or backward a series of from four to eight numbers, to subtract 7 serially from 100, to retell an anecdote, or to act adequately on a set of simple directions. Even when necessary, this portion of the examination may be so conducted that the patient need not resent or hardly be aware of the fact that he is being tested.

Mood and Emotional State: The fixity or range of the patient's conations and affects: e.g., indifference, anxiety, depression, euphoria, hostility, etc., will have been in part verbally communicated by him during the interview. In addition, the examiner may have noted such physiologic and mimetic accompaniments as flushings, lachrymation, pupillary dilations, tremors, jaw-clenchings and various muscular tensions, sudden startle reactions, and other visceral and motor expressions of emotion. The stooped posture, slow movements, low retarded speech and dolorous facies of the melancholic are especially noticeable; in such patients, the possibility of self-destructive preoccupations may be better investigated gently and indirectly (e.g., "are you sometimes so discouraged about your illness that you feel there is no use in going on?") than by direct questions as to frank plans for suicide. With empathy and experience the examiner will also more readily sense the touchy apprehensiveness of the anxiety neurotic, the bland ("*la belle indifference*") dependency of the so-called "conversion hysteric," the strained, restless, pseudoeuphoria of the hypomanic, the demanding, self-pitying, nihilistic attitudes of the depressive, or the dereistic, withdrawn distortions or deviant rapport of the schizoid or schizophrenic.

Preoccupations and Special Symptoms: When indicated, further inquiry may reveal persistent fantasies, significant dreams or nightmares, phobias, obsessive preoccupations, compulsions, hypochondriacal tendencies or fixations, diurnal or other variations in energy level or temperament, recurrent déjà-vu experiences, feelings of depersonalization, confusion or panic, transient absences or prolonged fugue states, etc. Even more serious psychological deviations may incidentally be uncovered, for instance: hallucinations may be described in response to an inquiry about "very vivid day-dreams or imagination," whereas paranoid or other delusions may emerge clearly (but should not be explicitly agreed to) during the interview.

Insight: This is always a complex, relative and variable aspect of the patient's past attitudes and current status. From a clinical standpoint, insight may be estimated along the following dimensions: (a) the patient's own explanations of his illness, (b) his ideas as to prognosis and treatment, and (c) the sincerity of his desires for, and cooperation with, medical and psychiatric therpy. However, the ostensible acceptance of the examiner's formulations by the patient should not necessarily be regarded as indicative of true understanding or impending behavioral change.

PSYCHIATRIC SIGNIFICANCE OF THE PHYSICAL EXAMINATION

The patient's conduct during this procedure, likewise, contributes evidence as to his mental status, e.g., excessive shyness, modesty, or exhibitionism; extreme passivity; suspiciousness or hypersensitiveness with regard to abdominal, vaginal or rectal examinations; irrational fear of transillumination or retinoscopy, and so on. Incidental observations should include the adequacy of oral, ungual, and other personal hygiene, tatoo marks, drug rashes, evidences of minor scarrings from repeated syncope, or signs of hypodermic or intravenous use of narcotics.

SUPPLEMENTARY PSYCHOLOGIC TESTING

Whenever there are difficulties in differential diagnosis or other special problems, the patient may be referred to a clinical psychologist for the following: (a) *Tests of intellectual functions*, such as the WAIS or the WISC, (b) *Tests of occupational preference or special abilities*, such as the Strong Vocational Guidance Scale, (c) *Personality tests* such as the "objective" Minnesota Multiphasic Personality Inventory (MMPI) and projective techniques such as the Rorschach and the Thematic Apperception, which can be the most revealing

ANCILLARY TECHNIQUES IN PSYCHIATRIC DIAGNOSIS

These include polygraphic recordings during questioning or history-taking ("lie detection"), hypnotic catharsis or regression, or the administration of drugs such as scopolamine ("truth serum") or intravenous sodium pentothal or sodium amytal. Such procedures are rarely if ever necessary in pyschiatric diagnosis and carry definite physical and psychologic dangers; however, the physician should be acquainted with their general significance. (See Masserman, J. H., "Practice of Dynamic Psychiatry," Chapter 4.)

PSYCHIATRIC FORMULATION

The formulation is designed to organize the information obtained during the psychiatric examination into a coherent and meaningful summary which has both explanatory and predictive value. From a formulation one can make inferences about diagnosis which then lead to statements about prognosis and the development of treatment plans for the patient. Importantly, the formulation serves the vital purpose of enabling the interviewer to order his own thinking about the patient into a logical sequence of meaningful and informative statements.

By definition, the task of comprehension involves reducing a mass of accumulated data from interviews, clinical examinations, and laboratory reports to a succinct group of statements which are selective and explanatory and which increase the clinician's and other's understanding of the patient.

When sufficient information has been gathered to make possible a comprehensive formulation, this should be integrated and summarized according to the following outline:

1. A brief description of the patient and his initial relationships to the examiner.

2. A succint statement of the precipitating circumstances, nature, duration, and course of the present illness.

3. An evaluation of organic factors as revealed by the medical history and by the physical, neurological, laboratory and other special examinations.

4. An analysis of constitutional and experiential vectors as indicated by the familial and personal history, and supplementary psychologic or other tests.

5. The current behavioral status as shown by direct psychiatric observation and ancillary nursing or other reports.

6. An interim diagnostic summary based on the above, including: (a) the presence and *relative prominence* of various psychiatric syndromes (e.g., anxiety, physiologic dysfunctions, depression, schizoid tendencies, etc.), (b) the relationship of these reactions to specific external stresses (environmental maladaptations) and (c) their roots in inner motivations, formative experiences and derived character patterns (psychodynamics).

7. Indications for further diagnostic procedures, medical or psychiatric.

8. Preliminary plans for therapy, as recorded under the following rubrics:

a. Immediate symptomatic relief by medication, sedation, physiotherapy, or other medical or surgical procedures.

b. Environmental alterations such as change of residence or work, or, if necessary, hospitalization for total care.

c. Projected nature and techniques of the psychotherapy to be employed.

d. Methods of securing the cooperation of the patient's friends and family in his treatment or, when necessary, in his legally arranged custodial care.

This formulation should be elaborated and amended as new facts become available, and supplemented by progress notes as the patient is treated and followed.

The above represents a fairly extended but by no means all-inclusive review of modern approaches to a comprehensive and dynamically oriented clinical examination.

CONDENSED SUMMARY

Since the symptomatology, course and therapy of every illness is influenced by the motivations, personality and environment of the patient, no comprehensive diagnosis or plan of therapy is complete without an adequate survey of these factors. As a final summary, the following may be copied for ready reference with proper sympathy and tact in actual clinical usage:

Psychiatric Survey

Neurotic Symptomatology: Determine the intensity and frequency of anxiety reactions, obsessive-phobic-compulsive states, hypomanic or depressive mood swings, disturbances of consciousness or motor control, drug intake, and recent impairments of intellectual functions and interpretations of reality.

Relationship to Environmental Stresses: Review the circumstances that precipitated, exacerbated or alleviated the above deviations in behavior and their accompanying organic (psychosomatic) dysfunctions, including the patient's reactions to previous examinations and therapy.

Personal History

Since normal and abnormal behavior can be best understood as an evolution of genetic, constitutional and adaptational patterns in relation to physical and emotional stresses, this section of the examination should comprise a pertinent review of the following data about the patient as a person:

Social History: Essential data about parents' occupations, educational levels, aspirations, values, and subcultural attitudes.

Family History: Brief descriptions of significant traits in parents, siblings or important relatives.

Birth and Early Development: Data on infantile traumata or illnesses, feeding disturbances, spasms, terrors, or other childhood neurotic tendencies.

Schooling and Early Socialization: Scholastic interests and performance, adjustments to discipline, and group participations.

Sexual Patterns: Marked deviations, special fears, and marital and parental adjustments.

Habits: Of food, sleep, recreation, and intake of alcohol, sedatives or other drugs.

Social Adjustments: Friendships, prejudices, hostilities, group participations, recreations, religious activities.

Occupational: Goals; level of initiative and performance; cooperation with employers, fellow and subordinates.

Military Service: Motivation and reactions in training or combat.

Previous Reactions to Injuries or Illnesses, including tendencies to emotional over-reactions, dependency litigations and invalidism.

Present Illness

Since the personal history is less a chronological account than a biographical review of the *origin and nature of the patient's characteristic patterns of conduct*, it will lead naturally into the circumstances that precipitated the present illness as previously surveyed.

The Current Behavioral ("Mental") Status

This consists of a summary of the patient's conduct as either directly observed during history-taking and physical examination, or as elicited by further inquiry. The data may be organized under the following headings:

General Behavior: Appearance, posture, mannerisms, dress, personal hygiene, etc.

Intellectual Level: As estimated from perceptive grasp, vocabulary, general information, logic and versatility of thought and cultural attainments.

Sensorium: Orientations: to time, space and identity; clarity of awareness and retention.

Mood and Emotional State: Excessive anxiety, euphoria, passivity, hostility, remoteness, indifference, etc. In melancholic patients the possibility of suicidal impulses is of immediate practical importance.

Special Symptoms: Such as hypochondriacal preoccupations; panic or fugue states; déjà-vu; clouded consciousness, etc.

Psychotic Manifestations: Affective distortions, hallucinations, bizarre fantastic preoccupations, grandiose or persecutory delusions and paranoid systematizations.

Insight: The patient's own concepts as to (a) the nature of his illness, (b) his ideas as to treatment and prognosis, (c) his cooperation with examination and therapy.

Formulation

The above information may be recorded or, in psychiatric consultation, more briefly appended to the medical or surgical record under the following headings:

Organic Factors in the present illness, as determined by the medical history and physical and laboratory findings.

Psychiatric and "Psychosomatic" Components of the current illness, and their predisposing and precipitating circumstances as determined by the psychiatric and personal history and mental status.

Indications for Further Diagnostic Procedures: medical, psychologic or special techniques.

Psychiatric Evaluation in Clinical and Prognostic Terms rather than in pejorative labels.

Therapy: Comprising methods of immediate systematic relief or environmental readjustments, need of hospitalization for special procedures, and plans for long-term medical and psychiatric treatment and eventual social rehabilitation.

REFERENCES

1. Freedman, A.M. and Kaplan, H. I.: *Interpreting Personality*. New York, Science House, 1973.
2. Gray, W., Duhl, F. J. and Rizzo N. D. (Eds.): *General Systems Theory and Psychiatry*. Boston, Little, Brown, 1969.
3. Spiegel, J.: *Transactions*. New York, Science House, 1972.
4. Weisman, A. D. The psychodynamic formulations of conflict. *Arch. Gen. Psychiat.* 1: 72–93, 288–309, 1959.

AUTHOR INDEX

SUBJECT INDEX